THE SELF-CARE
PRESCRIPTION

D1019216

The Self-Care Prescription *takes a smart, systematic, scientifically based approach to self-care, showing you how to enrich your life no matter what your circumstances may be. It offers a careful exploration of your needs and wishes, provides a host of creative new possibilities and choices, and gives gentle instructions for arranging your life in a way that is more in alignment with who you really are. Highly recommended!*

—**Christopher Germer, PhD**, author of *The Mindful Path to Self-Compassion*, coauthor of *Teaching the Mindful Self-Compassion Program*

Although it focuses on self-care, The Self-Care Prescription *is really a comprehensive guide to creating a full, vibrant, and healthy life. The book is structured so that each reader can create a personalized self-care plan, choosing the areas of life that matter most to them. I highly recommend this book to anyone who is ready to invest even a little bit of time and energy in themselves, and would like a supportive guide along the way.*

—**Melissa Platt, PhD**

The Self-Care Prescription *is a timely, practical, and much-needed resource for anyone who is feeling drained, overwhelmed, or anxious. Dr. Gobin provides practical steps anyone can take to better nourish their mind, body, and spirit. Her writing is refreshing, action-oriented, and compassionate as she lays out a roadmap to move us out of the stress zone and into more empowered lives.*

—**Thema Bryant-Davis, PhD**, author of *Thriving in the Wake of Trauma: A Multicultural Guide*

Self-care is one of the most important, yet often most neglected, tasks that we must embrace in order to live our richest, fullest, and healthiest lives. In The Self-Care Prescription, *Robyn Gobin clearly explains why self-care is critical, the costs of neglecting self-care, and most importantly, how you can take better care of yourself. With a kind, warm, and compassionate tone, Robyn takes care of you as you learn to take better care of yourself. I will be recommending and gifting this much-needed book to family, friends, and clients alike.*

—**Aisling Leonard-Curtin, MS**, chartered psychologist with the Psychological Society of Ireland, coauthor of *The Power of Small: Making Tiny but Powerful Changes When Everything Feels Too Much*

The Self-Care Prescription *is the ideal self-help book for learning to live a life full of growth and engagement. The book has thoughtful exercises, bringing to life the most personally relevant aspects of self-care.*

—Robyn Walser, PhD, author of *The Mindful Couple: How Acceptance and Mindfulness Can Lead to the Love You Want*

THE SELF-CARE PRESCRIPTION

Powerful Solutions to
Manage Stress, Reduce Anxiety
& Increase Well-Being

Robyn L. Gobin, PhD

ALTHEA
PRESS

To Korey and Justice for challenging me to become the best version of myself and filling my life with so much joy.

Copyright © 2019 by Althea Press, Emeryville, California

No part of this publication may be reproduced, stored in a retrieval system, or transmitted in any form or by any means, electronic, mechanical, photocopying, recording, scanning, or otherwise, except as permitted under Sections 107 or 108 of the 1976 United States Copyright Act, without the prior written permission of the Publisher. Requests to the Publisher for permission should be addressed to the Permissions Department, Althea Press, 6005 Shellmound Street, Suite 175, Emeryville CA 94608.

Limit of Liability/Disclaimer of Warranty: The Publisher and the author make no representations or warranties with respect to the accuracy or completeness of the contents of this work and specifically disclaim all warranties, including without limitation warranties of fitness for a particular purpose. No warranty may be created or extended by sales or promotional materials. The advice and strategies contained herein may not be suitable for every situation. This work is sold with the understanding that the Publisher is not engaged in rendering medical, legal, or other professional advice or services. If professional assistance is required, the services of a competent professional person should be sought. Neither the Publisher nor the author shall be liable for damages arising herefrom. The fact that an individual, organization, or website is referred to in this work as a citation and/ or potential source of further information does not mean that the author or the Publisher endorses the information the individual, organization, or website may provide or recommendations they/it may make. Further, readers should be aware that websites listed in this work may have changed or disappeared between when this work was written and when it is read.

For general information on our other products and services or to obtain technical support, please contact our Customer Care Department within the United States at (866) 744-2665, or outside the United States at (510) 253-0500.

Althea Press publishes its books in a variety of electronic and print formats. Some content that appears in print may not be available in electronic books, and vice versa.

TRADEMARKS: Althea Press and the Althea Press logo are trademarks or registered trademarks of Callisto Media Inc. and/or its affiliates, in the United States and other countries, and may not be used without written permission. All other trademarks are the property of their respective owners. Althea Press is not associated with any product or vendor mentioned in this book.

Interior and Cover Designer: Michael Cook
Editor: Camille Hayes
Production Editor: Erum Khan

ISBN: Print 978-1-64152-393-6 | eBook 978-1-64152-394-3

CONTENTS

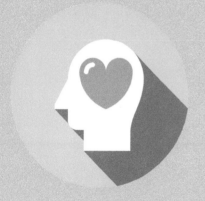

CHAPTER 1

Why You Should Care About Self-Care

Oh, you know, I'm okay. I'm busy and I haven't slept in weeks, but I'm making it. This was the response a coworker gave me when I asked how she was doing a few years back. This response has stuck with me, because I think it rings true for many of us. In my years as a therapist, I've heard clients express similar feelings, and I have certainly felt that way in my own life at times. Like a worn-out T-shirt, our various responsibilities have pulled us in so many different directions that we end up stretched way too thin; we're threadbare, with little to nothing of value left to give ourselves. We dream of escaping to sandy beaches and clear waters, but the time never seems to be right to take a vacation. We wear many hats—parent, worker, spouse, son or daughter, sibling, student, and the list goes on. Each of these hats demands a certain level of time, money, and energy that slowly depletes us from day to day.

Self-Care Is Fundamental

Self-care is in the air these days. You've probably seen a thousand posts about it on social media and heard the familiar phrase dropped in advertisements. Self-care is offered as a remedy for virtually everything. It's a popular recommendation from nearly everyone—from doctors and bloggers to life coaches and therapists. With most self-care advice, you might be encouraged to get a mani-pedi, treat yourself to a nice meal, take an exotic vacation, or take a long, hot bath. Everyone's telling you to *take time for yourself,* but aside from pampering yourself and "me time," what is self-care and why is it so important?

Simply put, self-care means taking care of yourself. But that means more than just treating yourself to occasional luxuries; it means taking responsibility for your well-being in all the import-ant areas of your life. It involves spending dedicated time getting to know who you are and what you need, and then committing to giving yourself what you need to be happy, healthy, and fully present for your life.

When we allow our family, job, and other responsibilities to consume all our time and attention—without spending resources on ourselves—we end up physically exhausted, emotionally dis-connected from ourselves and our loved ones, and (despite having a whole 24 hours to work with each day) always short on time. When we have the audacity to take a break from it all, we feel guilty, things fall through the cracks, or we just can't seem to stop thinking about all the items that are piling up on our to-do list while we're suppos-edly relaxing.

Before we know it, we can find ourselves living a life we don't even recognize. We get so consumed by work and responsibilities that there is no time for connection with friends, pursuing our dreams, rest, or intimacy with our family and partners. Day in and day out, we go through the motions, crossing items off the to-do list; all the while, we're overcommitted, unhappy, and unfulfilled. We feel pow-erless, as if we're just passengers along for the ride. We've forgotten how powerful we can be and how much control we have in determining the course of our own lives.

And so, when someone asks how we're doing, we might find ourselves replying, like my coworker: "I'm okay, just making it." But here's the thing: I want more for you than just "okay." I want you to feel confident, energized, motivated, and empowered. I want you to play an active role in determining the direction your life is headed. That's why I decided to write this book—to remind you, and all of us, that we can *choose*. You can begin again anytime you want and forge a new life path. You can take the wheel and change the course of your life. Yes, things will be hard sometimes. But, in the midst of it all, I never want you to forget about yourself and your needs. Taking care of *you* is the best thing you can do for your job, your family, and your friends. Self-care is essential not just for feeling good but also for functioning well in everyday life.

I want to make it clear from the beginning that self-care is *not* just about feeling good. Sure, much of what you do for self-care will bring you pleasure, but this will not always be the case. Simply put, self-care is not always fun or relaxing, and you won't always "feel like" doing it. Sometimes self-care involves forgiving yourself for past mistakes, setting boundaries in relationships, making that medical or dental appointment you've been putting off, saying no to a fun night out because you're sleep deprived, or choosing to walk away from a job or a relationship you have outgrown.

Self-care is about making yourself a priority, whatever your life circumstances. Self-care is, fundamentally, about bringing balance back to a life that has grown imbalanced from too many commitments or responsibilities.

How Do You "Do" Self-Care?

The popular idea of self-care often shown in magazines, blogs, and TV news segments typically includes ice cream, bubble baths, massages, or pedicures. While these kinds of "me time," "Treat Yo' Self" strategies can play a role in a self-care routine, real self-care is a much more substantive, holistic endeavor, touching every aspect of a person's life. So, truly taking care of your own needs requires not just scheduling fun activities now and then, but also doing some self-reflection to see how things stand in your life, where you most want or need to make change, and how best to bring those changes about. Self-care is about taking a serious look in the mirror and making changes that will give your life more balance, meaning, purpose, and fulfillment.

Let's say, for example, you've been battling chronic pain, anxiety, or depression silently for months, but you have not noticed any significant improvement. Self-care in this situation might involve being honest with yourself about your pain and your difficulty managing it on your own, and then taking the vulnerable step of reaching out to a doctor or therapist for help. This can be hard, because so many of us have bought into the idea that we are somehow weak if we're unable to solve problems on our own. Nothing could be further from the truth. In a society that glorifies self-reliance, it takes a lot of strength to ask for help when you need it. This process of learning to truly take care of yourself might not always be pleasurable, and you may encounter some mental roadblocks that you'll need to overcome, but it is self-care nonetheless.

What This Book Offers

I'll tell you what I tell my clients: I'm not a miracle worker. Neither is this book. I wish I had a magic wand that could take away all your emotional pain and fix all the problems you are facing this very moment, but that simply isn't possible. I don't have all the answers, but what I do have is knowledge and a proven set of skill-building strategies that I believe will help you create the life you desire, brick by brick. I'll be right there alongside you as you put in the effort and hard work to bring about the changes you most want to see in your life. It will require openness on your part; if you stick with me and implement the tips and techniques I suggest here, I am confident that you'll walk away from this experience equipped with the tools you need to continue along your self-care journey, more clearheaded and empowered than when you began.

This book is structured around the six essential dimensions of wellness as defined by the National Wellness Institute: the physical, spiritual, emotional, intellectual, vocational, and social domains. Self-care is about more than looking and feeling good; it involves nurturing every aspect of yourself—mind, body, and spirit. I like to think of the dimensions of wellness like a car. Each part of a car plays a vital role in the overall functioning of the vehicle. If any part of the car is broken or malfunctioning—for example, the brakes wear out—the car becomes unstable, and it cannot function the way it was intended to. Sure, you can continue to drive your car when your brakes need work, but eventually you'll run the risk of doing serious damage to yourself and your car.

Like a car in need of work, we can "get by" and still function while only attending to some dimensions of wellness, but that choice comes with downsides. To ensure that we keep running smoothly we need periodic tune-ups, and we'd be wise not to ignore any warning signals that an area of our life needs attention. Just like we wouldn't purchase a brand-new car and drive it around for years without ever taking it in for routine oil changes and maintenance, our bodies, minds, and spirits require the same level of upkeep. Let's quickly review what each dimension of wellness entails.

Physical: Physical wellness is all about how your body functions. To function optimally, your body needs proper nourishment, exercise, and healthy habits.

Social: We were created for social connection. We are at our best when we have healthy relationships with people who genuinely care about us, respect us, and lift us up.

Intellectual: Just like your body needs exercise, so does your brain! You're never too old to grow and learn something new. Intellectual wellness is all about engaging in activities that feed your creativity and keep your mind sharp.

Vocational: Life is too short to be doing work that doesn't make you feel good. Vocational self-care involves finding meaning in the work you do and knowing how to cope when you find yourself in a less than optimal employment situation.

Spiritual: When we are spiritually healthy, we realize that we exist beyond the physical and our life has a sense of meaning and purpose.

Emotional: Oh, feelings. When they're unpleasant, we feel like we can't live with them, and when they're pleasant, we definitely wouldn't want to survive without them. The truth is, we were meant to experience a range of emotions—both pleasure and pain. Emotional wellness is all about embracing your full emotional experience and having skills that help you cope when emotions are painful and intense.

Each of the following six chapters begins with a general discussion of what's important about that particular self-care domain and what's needed for that domain to stay healthy and well balanced. Then, I'll make it personal by leading you in discussions and activities that will help you create a vision for how you want to show up in your life around each area of wellness. I'll also share proven mind-set strategies and techniques that will propel you toward your personal goals in each category.

Every exercise I offer can be tailored to meet your specific circumstances and life demands. This is about incorporating self-care into your life in a way that works for you. There are no one-size-fits-all methods over here! As you read through the strategies, I encourage you to think outside the box and find creative ways to make each strategy your own.

Finding What Works for You

By now you've probably got the idea: This book covers a lot! Because every self-care domain plays a critical role in achieving the balance you need, you'll benefit from working on all six domains. However, if you came to this book with a particular problem in mind—say, feeling stuck in your professional life—feel free to go directly to chapter 5, which focuses on vocational self-care, and begin there. But don't shortchange yourself! Plan to work on all the chapters eventually, because all the skills and exercises in this book build on and reinforce one another.

Not every recommendation will work the same way for everyone. This book is jam-packed with powerful exercises, tools, and techniques so that, whatever your circumstances, you can find something that works for you. I do recommend that you try everything at least once. Once you've done that, feel free to take the techniques that are a good fit for you and leave behind things that were less useful. This is all about you upgrading your life in a way that is manageable and sustainable in the long run.

Let's Get Started

My sincere hope is that you will walk away from this book with skills that equip you to prioritize your health and happiness despite the challenges and complexities that life throws your way. Bottom line: I want to help you live your best life. This book offers proven-effective techniques to help you integrate self-care strategies into your life. But as author John C. Maxwell said, "Dreams don't work unless you do."

I believe you have the potential to create a life where you not only look good, but you also feel good. So many of us have perfected the art of looking good. We have become pros at wearing the "I'm okay" mask. Our outsides are dressed up nicely—stylish clothes, pretty smiles, positive attitudes—but inside, things aren't so pretty. We've stopped enjoying life, we crave deeper connection, and we've lost ourselves in the process of taking care of everyone else. This is your invitation to put *you* first. It's time to stop waiting for "someday." Learn how to take better care of yourself *today*.

It is possible to be an incredible partner, parent, friend, and/or family member, and still take care of yourself. I will show you how. Some of the strategies may be familiar to you, and others may feel new and different. When you hear something that is familiar or "tried and true" for you, challenge yourself to look at that skill with new eyes. There are three things you will need to get the most out of this book: an open mind, a pen, and a notebook. As you move through the book, I encourage you to use the notebook for journaling, list-making, and planning how you will implement various recommendations. Commit to setting aside as much time daily or weekly as you can to read this book and practice the strategies within. Part of what this book will teach you is how to carve out time for yourself, so it's okay to start small. You can't make over your life overnight. Just start.

Here is my goal for you: By the time you reach the end of this book, you will be experiencing so many benefits from taking care of yourself that you'll want to maximize self-care time in your schedule. Are you ready to start? Let's go! I'll be rooting for you.

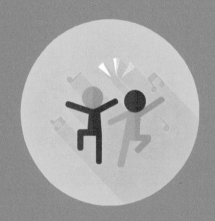

CHAPTER 2

Friends, Family & Fun
Social Self-Care

START HERE IF

Start with social self-care if you want to:

- → Improve the quality of your relationships
- → Revive your social life
- → Spend free time engaged with people and in activities that energize and recharge you
- → Find more time for recreation and play
- → Engage in hobbies that are fun, fulfilling, and improve your overall health

Your Social Needs

We're hardwired for social connection. From the time we exit the womb, we are motivated to communicate and form relationships with others. Due to our limited physical abilities at birth, as infants we come into the world equipped with sophisticated social intelligence that allows us to communicate, understand social cues, and shape our behavior in ways that maximize the chances we'll get our basic needs for food, clothing, belonging, and shelter met. When we mature and gain independence, our need for social connection can take a back seat to other demands of adult life. As our days become filled with work, bills, and family responsibilities, we find less and less time for social self-care.

Social self-care can be defined as nurturing your need for connection with other people. It involves taking care of existing relationships and friendships, creating new connections, and establishing boundaries in relationships with others so that those connections stay healthy. Social self-care is important because it fosters belongingness and connectedness. *Belongingness* is an innate human need to be an accepted member of a group (for example, family, friends, and coworkers, and/or organized group activities such as teams, sports, classes, or trivia nights) or to be a part of something bigger than yourself (for example, volunteering, charitable contributions or activities, and humanitarian efforts). *Social connectedness* is our experience of how close we are to other people.

Research has found that social connections are good for our mental health. On the other hand, a lack of social connection is associated with poorer health, greater stress, and feelings of loneliness, depression, anxiety, and guilt. Social self-care through frequent contact with friends, family activities, hobbies, and organized group activities increases the chances we will be happy, healthy, and well adjusted.

What Do You Want from Your Social Life?

An important place to start improving your social self-care is to create a vision for yourself. This is a one-sentence statement of what you want your social life to be like. Once you're clear on that, you can begin taking positive steps in that direction. Your social self-care vision should make you feel excited about leveling up your social life. In creating your vision, also consider *why* you want your social life to change in those ways. Ask yourself, "Why is it important to me to be social? What do I gain from making time for social self-care?" Identifying personal reasons why social self-care is important in your life can motivate you to make it more of a priority, even when other commitments seem more pressing.

Here are some questions to guide you in creating a personal social self-care vision and discovering your "why." Get out your notebook, and as you're answering the questions, challenge yourself to go beyond simply thinking about this as an intellectual exercise. Give yourself permission to get creative. Engage all your senses. Create a vivid, detailed mental image of what your future social self-care looks like: Who and what do you see? What do you taste? What smells are present? What emotions do you feel?

Making Social Self-Care a Reality

- **What kind of friend would you like to be?** How do you want to feel when you are with your friends? What would you need to do differently to feel the way you want to feel?
- **What kind of romantic partner would you like to be?** How do you want to feel when you are with your romantic partner? What would you need to do differently to feel the way you want to feel?
- **What kind of employer or employee would you like to be?** How do you want to feel when you are working with others? What would you need to do differently to feel the way you want to feel?
- **What kind of family member (e.g., parent, grandparent, child, sibling, cousin, aunt or uncle, etc.) would you like to be?** How do you want to feel when you are with your family members? What would you need to do differently to feel the way you want to feel?
- **When was the last time you felt engaged, excited, safe, and supported in your social life?** What were you doing? Who were you with? What would need to happen to recreate this scenario?
- **Describe your ideal social life.** What kind of people do you want to be spending time with? How do you want to feel when you are

living your ideal social life? What would you be doing differently to feel the way you want to feel?

- **If you had "free time" where you were feeling rested and energized, what types of activities would you like to engage in with others?** Why? How do you want to feel during your free time? What would you need to do differently to feel the way you want to feel?

- **What types of group-related hobbies do you have?** How do those hobbies make you feel when you are participating in them? What new hobbies (if any) are you interested in exploring in a group setting? How do you want to feel when you are participating in hobbies? What would you need to do differently to feel the way you want to feel?

Your Social Self-Care Vision

In your notebook, try your hand at crafting your own social self-care vision. It doesn't have to be long, just a sentence or two. Here's an example: *"I am shaping relationships in which deep connection is plentiful, love and respect is mutual, and contact is pleasant and consistent."*

Your Social Self-Care "Why"

Complete this sentence: *Social self-care is important to me because . . .*

Engage

Now that you've started to develop a personal vision for social self-care, it's time to make your vision a reality. In our busy lives, we have legitimate obligations—like family, work, and chores—that can take up a good portion of the day and leave us feeling like we don't have time for socializing. However, it can also be that you aren't prioritizing your social life because you feel wary of reengaging socially. For example, if you've experienced a painful breakup, it's normal to be skeptical about starting a new relationship. The same thing goes for friends and family. When you've been hurt in past relationships, it's normal to want to avoid getting close to people so that you don't get hurt again.

Once we've put our social lives on the back burner, it can become the "new normal" for us. Even though we desire social connection, we feel more comfortable being alone because it feels safer. We might find ourselves getting comfortable with infrequent or inconsistent social contact. So how do we begin to create a habit of social self-care that will last?

Where to Start:
Create a Social Self-Care Plan

Spend some time getting clear on what you would like to do and who you would like to do that activity with. Grab your notebook and take the following steps:

1. List your favorite things to do. Circle one activity you'd like to pursue in the next month.

2. List the people with whom you would like to engage in that activity.

3. Looking at this month's calendar, select two or three dates and times you would be willing to set aside for this activity.

4. Reach out to the people on your list. You may choose to reach out by text, e-mail, social-media messenger, or with a phone call. Share the potential activity and the dates and times that work for your schedule, and ask if they might be interested and available to join you.

5. Once they respond, determine what is needed to set the activity up for success. For example, if you are having dinner, are reservations needed? If yes, go ahead and make those reservations.

6. Troubleshoot challenges and barriers. If you do not receive a response after a day or so, try not to take it personally. Just like you have obligations that have kept you away from engaging socially, so do your family, friends, partners, and

acquaintances. Extend them some grace. Try a different method of contact.

7. Be flexible. If none of the people you reached out to are available on your desired dates and times, consider alternate dates or inviting different people. If that does not work or the people you intended to spend time with have to cancel plans, consider engaging in the activity alone. You never know who you might meet when you are willing to show up!

If you had difficulty with step one or two, reread your responses to the questions and prompts in "What Do You Want from Your Social Life?" (see page 12) to guide you in creating this plan. Which listed activities or people excite you the most? Use these as a starting point, and later, when you're ready, try some of the other activities you listed and invite some different people to join you.

Try Something New: Think Creatively

Sometimes your social self-care can benefit from trying something you've never done before. It's a great way to make lasting memories and potentially create new social connections. The following questions and suggestions can get your creative juices flowing:

- What new activity, food, or venue have you been wanting to visit or try that you just haven't had time for?
- When do you feel most adventurous and willing to try something new—particular days of the week, times of the day, after checking a major task off your to-do list . . . ?
- Ask a close friend, family member, or coworker what they enjoy doing in their free time. If it sounds interesting, consider trying their favorite activity on for size.
- Visit your local city's events page and browse local upcoming events. Take note of what stands out to you.
- Search your city on Meetup.com or a similar Internet service to find new activities that interest you and meet people who share similar interests.

Making the Time: Prioritize Social Plans

Two of the most common excuses I hear (and have used myself!) when trying to make space for socializing is "I don't have time" and "I don't have the energy." The truth is, we *do* have time and energy for the things that matter most to us. It's a matter of making social self-care a priority just like you prioritize work, school, or parenting.

One of the best strategies for making time to socialize is to schedule it on your calendar. The key here is to choose a social activity you really enjoy, plan to do it with people you genuinely like to spend time with, and select a time when you're likely to have energy and minimal distractions. Whether you use an electronic calendar or a physical one, block out time in your schedule, and then guard this time just as you would a job obligation or an important medical appointment.

At the same time, remember to be flexible. If something comes up that you absolutely cannot avoid—for instance, you get the flu or there's a family emergency—accept the reality of the situation, *and* be sure to reschedule your social plans so that you get in the habit of making this time a priority.

Play

Play for adults has gotten a bad rap in our society. When we think of playing, we imagine toys, sandboxes, and swing sets—in other words, childish things that don't play a role in adult life. Play and recreation are typically regarded as activities solely for young children, but this is a very limited concept of play. Play and recreation involve complete immersion in voluntary activities for the sole purpose of simply *enjoying yourself*. (Sounds radical, I know!)

Play can include a wide variety of activities ranging from sports and vigorous exercise to dancing or playing a board game with friends. Just as play is healthy and stimulating for children, play has been found to have health benefits for adults, including reduced levels of stress and anxiety, enhanced creativity and innovation, better sleep, greater feelings of relaxation, improved heart and lung functioning, and lower risk for ailments like cancer and diabetes.

So, how do we build healthy recreation into our busy lives? The good news is, the possibilities are nearly endless when it comes to the type of recreation you can choose. Below are some ideas of how you might incorporate more play into your life. As you read through these suggestions, jot down some ideas for implementing them in your notebook.

- **Incorporate recreation into your daily routine.** Recreation in daily life can take the form of listening to music, learning a new language, solving puzzles, exercising, swimming, hiking, and setting aside time to take a walk or play with your pet, partner, or children. List some ways you can incorporate recreation into your daily routine.

- **Play with a group.** You can play a board game, video game, or team-based card game; play along with others while you watch a TV game show; watch funny videos together; or enjoy the challenge of an escape room with a group of family and/or friends. (Escape rooms are themed adventure games in which players are given a set amount of time to work as a team to solve puzzles, riddles, and secret codes.) List some of your favorite games in these categories that you'd like to try with family and/or friends.

- **Incorporate play at work.** Ideas for play at work include taking a lunchtime walk with colleagues, sharing a fun story or pictures from your family's latest adventure, or chatting with a coworker about a shared interest. Many companies have team-building activities that involve play. For example, one of my previous employers had quarterly team-building days where we would all take the afternoon off from work to do fun things like playing laser tag or simply getting to know each other on a deeper level over a leisurely meal. Periodically, my husband and his colleagues create fun games and prizes to reward members of their sales team for achieving a high sales volume. Whatever you choose, the goals of the activity should be to have fun, communicate, get creative, and build deeper, more meaningful connections.

Unwind

Adult life is stressful. Whether or not we know it, we could all stand to decompress from the pressure we feel all day—we function better and we're easier to be around when we take time to unwind. Social self-care is most effective when we're attuned to our needs, feelings, thoughts, and desires. This kind of attunement requires us to pause and pay attention to what we are experiencing in the moment. In our fast-paced society where we are constantly bombarded with people, things, and environmental demands that are all equally vying for our time and attention, it can be a revolutionary act to intentionally pause and allow our own needs to rise to the top of the list. When we take the time to unwind, we're more available and open to spending time with other people.

Mindfulness is one way to unwind from the stress of "adulting." Mindfulness involves slowing down and purposefully paying attention to our moment-to-moment experience in a particular way. When we're being mindful, we allow thoughts, feelings, and bodily sensations to be just as they are—without trying to change them or wishing they were different. When we are attuned to our moment-to-moment experience, we come to know ourselves more intimately, and we notice that our thoughts, feelings, and sensations are constantly shifting and changing. Because judgments and labels of our experience as "good" or "bad" can result in unnecessary pain and suffering, mindfulness invites us to release them.

Why might mindfulness practice be beneficial for unwinding? Practicing a mindfulness technique such as breath awareness meditation activates the body system that calms and relaxes us. It allows us to be more aware of what is actually happening in the here and now. When we are calm and present, we're much better able to listen to what we need and want as it relates to social self-care, and we're poised to make choices that align with our social self-care vision. The following exercises will guide you in practicing mindfulness as a way to unwind and relax.

This short breathing exercise can easily be incorporated into your day. It is designed to help you unwind and ground you in the present moment. By paying attention to your breath, you can help your body relax. Note that the recommended times here are approximate, but set a timer for the full five minutes before you begin so you can take full advantage of your relaxation time.

1. **Sit in a chair with a straight back and relaxed posture.** Allow your hands to rest softly on your lap. Allow your body to be fully supported by the chair, releasing any tension and letting your leg and thigh muscles relax with your feet pressed into the floor.

2. **Close your eyes, or lower your eyelids halfway, and focus your vision on a single spot five feet in front of you.** This step helps relax your mind, reduce distractions, and focus your attention on your internal experience.

3. **For the next minute and a half, take note of your internal experience.** What sounds do you hear? What bodily sensations are making themselves known? What emotions are present? What thoughts are in your mind?

4. **Make space for whatever you notice, regardless of whether it is pleasurable, uncomfortable, or middle-of-the-road.** Mindfulness invites you to accept your experience as it is without trying to change it or wishing it were different. You are not looking for anything in particular. Simply notice and observe your experience as it unfolds moment to moment with gentleness, with curiosity, and without judgment.

5. **For the next two minutes, shift your focus to the physical sensations of breathing.** One way to locate the physical sensations of your body as you breathe is to pay attention

to the rise and the fall of your belly. As you breathe in, notice how your belly expands. And, as you breathe out, notice how your belly contracts. You may find it easiest to make contact with the physical sensations of breathing in your nostrils or chest. Allow your attention to rest wherever in your body it's easiest for you to feel the sensations. Challenge yourself to pay attention to the inhalation in its entirety; be present with it until it transitions into an exhalation. Then pay attention to the whole exhalation until it turns into an inhalation.

6. **Do not try to change or modify the pattern of your breathing.** Simply observe the breath with gentleness and curiosity. Allow it to ground you in the here and now. Breathe in. Breathe out. Be present with each breath from moment to moment, as best as you can.

7. **For the remaining minute and a half, expand your attention from the breath and become aware of your entire body as a whole.** Notice the body sitting here breathing from head to toe. Pay attention to physical sensations that are present on the outer surface of the body at the skin, as well as those sensations arising from inside the body. Notice sensations that are pleasurable. Also notice any discomfort or tension that is present, as well as those sensations that are neutral (neither pleasurable nor uncomfortable). Gently explore all sensations with openness and curiosity. Take in all sensations as they are.

8. **Conclude the exercise and open your eyes.**

Because this exercise takes only a few minutes, you can do it several times throughout the day to bring yourself a sense of peace and calmness. This five-minute breathing break may be just what you need to appreciate more fully the time you spend with others.

It's hard to unwind when you're walking around feeling tense. Often-times we unknowingly hold tension and stress in our muscles. This progressive muscle relaxation exercise is designed to help you learn the difference between a tensed and relaxed muscle. It will also teach you how to relax your muscles.

Starting at your toes, this exercise invites you to gradually work your way up the body, tightening and then relaxing each major muscle group. You will tighten each muscle group for about 15 seconds, then release the contraction and focus on the sensation of each relaxed muscle for 15 seconds. Take time to notice the changes you feel when a muscle group is relaxed versus when it is tense.

Progressive muscle relaxation is best performed seated or lying down on a flat surface in a quiet, distraction-free place. You may practice progressive muscle relaxation as often as you like to support relaxation. Be careful when tensing your muscles. If you feel intense pain while completing this exercise, you may be tensing too hard. It is best to gently tense your muscles. Consult your physician if you have any medical conditions that might hinder physical activity. Use the following script to guide yourself through this exercise:

- **Feet:** Curl your toes. Hold; then relax.
- **Calves:** Squeeze your calf muscles by flexing your toes upward toward your shins. Hold; then relax.
- **Thighs:** Squeeze your thigh muscles. Hold; then relax.
- **Buttocks:** Clench your buttocks. Hold; then relax.
- **Stomach:** Suck in your stomach. Hold; then relax.
- **Chest:** Breathe in deeply. Hold; then relax.
- **Back:** Arch your back. Hold; then relax.
- **Arms:** Make fists and tighten your biceps by bending your arm at the elbow and bringing your forearm up toward your shoulder. Hold; then relax.
- **Hands:** Make fists. Hold; then relax.
- **Neck and Shoulders:** Lift your shoulders up toward your ears. Hold; then relax.

- **Mouth**: Clench your teeth together, noticing the strain on your jaw. Hold; then relax.
- **Eyes**: Close your eyes tightly. Hold; then relax.
- **Forehead**: Raise your eyebrows as high as you can. Hold; then relax.

You might find it helpful to listen to an audio recording of someone guiding you through the steps of progressive muscle relaxation. This allows you to focus fully on the physical sensations of tensing and relaxing your muscles. There are many free audio recordings available on YouTube and smartphone apps. One progressive muscle relaxation audio recording I recommend is from the Dartmouth Student Wellness Center website (see page 137). Again, if you have any preexisting medical conditions that could be worsened by tensing your muscles, for your health and comfort I recommend consulting with your medical doctor before engaging in this exercise.

Reward Yourself

Building new habits isn't easy. It takes time and consistency to see benefits. To keep yourself motivated, reward yourself along the way to building your new habit. Just as you might reward your dog for "pot-tying" outside (as opposed to on the carpet), you can treat yourself to something special after engaging in a particular social self-care activity, which will motivate you to continue prioritizing social self-care. Here are some ways you might choose to treat yourself for following through on your plans:

- Buy yourself a new gadget, book, or clothing item.
- Watch your favorite movie.
- Take a relaxing bath.
- Go for a massage.
- Listen to music you enjoy.

Nurture

As we grow older and our responsibilities increase, we spend less and less time on our friendships. Similarly, our romantic relationships can become less of a priority when the honeymoon phase is over and we get busy with work and/or children. In the same way, our family relationships can grow distant if we are not intentional about nurturing those bonds. To stay healthy and connected, our relationships need ongoing attention and care. This relationship "maintenance" involves spending quality time together, doing fun shared activities, and expressing gratitude for actions and qualities we appreciate.

Studies show that supportive, healthy relationships provide positive health benefits and can serve as a buffer against stress and mental health challenges. Given the importance of relationships to overall health and wellness, it is important to understand the qualities of a healthy relationship. Take a look.

Identify the Qualities of Healthy Relationships

How do you know whether your relationships are healthy or unhealthy? Use the following checklist to examine the health and quality of your current relationships. In your notebook, answer yes or no for each relationship you are examining. Each "yes" answer signals an aspect that is beneficial to the health of the relationship.

1. You enjoy open and clear communication.

2. You communicate frequently.

3. You both feel loved and respected, even during disagreements.

4. You support each other.

5. You have the ability to solve disagreements in a manner that is respectful and pleasing to both of you.

6. You feel physically safe with each other.

7. You feel comfortable being your authentic selves around each other.

8. You are both comfortable expressing your honest opinions and feelings around each other.

9. You are comfortable making requests of each other.

10. You are both comfortable saying no or expressing an opposing opinion.

11. You each make voluntary sacrifices for the good of the relationship.

12. There is an absence of physical violence (e.g., hitting, beating, choking, burning, pinching, slapping, punching, grabbing, biting, pushing, shoving, or otherwise causing harm to you or your family, pets, children, or belongings).

13. There is an absence of sexual abuse or coercion (e.g., fondling or unwanted sexual touching, insisting on sex despite victim's objections, penetration of victim's body against their will, attempted rape, coercion).

14. There is an absence of emotional abuse (e.g., verbal insults, name-calling, manipulation, threats, swearing, yelling).

15. There is an absence of criticism or mistreatment on the basis of gender, ethnicity, religious beliefs, political beliefs, sexual orientation, ability status, nation of origin, or other personal attributes.

16. There is an absence of prior betrayal and/or infidelity.

17. You take an interest in each other's lives.

18. You each have interests and friends outside of the relationship.

19. You encourage interests and friendships outside of the relationship.

20. You consistently spend time together.

In your notebook, reflect on what you learned about the health of your relationships with family, friends, and partners. Revisit your social self-care vision. What aspects of your relationships do you want to focus on improving? What do your responses tell you about the extent to which your needs are currently being met in your relationships?

Revitalize Old Relationships

Back when I was a Girl Scout, we used to sing a song that went, "Make new friends, but keep the old. One is silver and the other is gold." Sometimes, our *gold* relationships need to be revitalized. They can get lost in the shuffle of daily life or taken for granted. What can you do to strengthen those long-standing, golden relationships? Grab your notebook and take the following steps:

1. **Identify one relationship to work toward reviving.** Why do you want to reconnect with this person in particular?

2. **Consider whether this relationship aligns with your social self-care vision.** Is this a person you feel good around? Do they value you, your time, and your perspective?

3. **What led you to neglect this relationship?** If betrayal, violence, or harm was the cause of the relationship going stale, consider whether it is in your best interest to reestablish this relationship. If you decide that rekindling this relationship is in your mutual best interest, reach out to that person.

4. **Don't take it personally if you don't get a response right away.** Check in after a few days have passed if they do not respond. Be flexible and open to a variety of responses. Some people may be willing to pick up where you left off. Others may not be interested in reconnecting at all. Still others may be slow to warm up to you, particularly if the relationship lag was due in large part to your neglect. Be willing to take responsibility for your role in the current status of the relationship. Be open to hearing their perspective and demonstrate respect for their feelings.

5. **Follow through and be patient.** Rebuilding an old relationship can be risky for some people.

6. **Take time to reflect on what you like about the person, and express gratitude and appreciation for their positive qualities and supportive behaviors.** When you are spending time with them, give them the gift of your attention to communicate that you value their companionship.

Keep in mind that the relationship you wish to rekindle may not turn out as you hope it will. Regardless of the outcome, you were courageous in going after something you wanted. Be kind to yourself by acknowledging and appreciating your own efforts.

Making New Friends

As you know, friendship is essential to our overall health and happiness, but making friends as an adult is no easy feat. Here is a list of strategies for meeting new people:

- **Intentionally place yourself in environments where like-minded people gather.** If your faith is important to you, join a congregation or group. If health and wellness are priorities in your life, join your local gym, yoga studio, or YMCA. If you love to read, attend an upcoming event at your local bookstore. Do a little research to find out where people who have similar interests hang out, and get involved.
- **Don't underestimate small talk.** Small talk allows you to get acquainted with people you do not know very well. Because the topics are less personal, it is a low-risk, high-reward situation. Some topics to consider include the weather, work/career interests, movies you've seen or books you've read, favorite foods, and observations about recent changes in your neighborhood.
- **Say yes to social invitations.** You never know who you might meet at an after-work happy hour or weekend barbecue.
- **Get to know your coworkers outside of work.** Organize a gathering of your colleagues outside of typical working hours.

- **Go to local events in your community.** Grab (or google!) the local newspaper and explore the lifestyle section or events calendar.
- **Try a new hobby.** Think back to what you liked to do as a child. Maybe you liked to dance or draw. Whatever your childhood passion was, find a class you can take that relates to it. Not only will you be doing something you enjoy, you'll meet new people who enjoy it, too.

Regardless of which strategies you try to make new friends, you'll need to risk some discomfort. Open yourself up to the endless possibilities that could unfold if you're willing to take even the smallest step outside your comfort zone.

Grow

Implementing your social self-care plan can be rewarding, but you might run into challenges along the way. These will come in two main forms: mental roadblocks and conflict. The following exercises will help you meet these challenges and set up an accountability plan, increasing your chances of making your social self-care vision a reality.

Often, when we dare to jump outside of our comfort zone and try something new, the greatest barrier can be our own mind. Worry, anxiety, and fear show up, creating mental roadblocks between us and our goals. If we are not careful, these thoughts can keep us from meaningful and fulfilling social lives. The good news is, you can choose to pursue your social self-care vision despite these negative feelings. You do not have to wait for them to go away before you take action. Your fear, anxiety, and worry are temporary thoughts and feelings based on judgments and predictions about the future—but these judgments and predictions are not always accurate.

Social Predictions and Mental Roadblocks

Forecasters use the science of meteorology, satellites, and computer programs to predict what the weather will be like each day. Although these predictions are sometimes correct, they can go very wrong. In fact, weather forecasts that attempt to predict the weather at 10 or more days out are accurate only 50 percent of the time. This is due, in large part, to the constant changing nature of the world's atmosphere. Similarly, your anxiety, worry, and fears try to predict the future, but they do so with even less accuracy than weather forecasters.

Grab your notebook, create a grid, and explore the accuracy of these feelings as shown in this example:

Predictions my worry, fears, and anxiety have made about relationships and social situations in the past:	Approximately how many times has my mind made this negative prediction in the last week?	How many times has the prediction been accurate?
They are going to think I'm stupid.	25	0—No one has ever said I'm stupid even when they disagreed with me.
I can't show weakness in relationships. I have to be strong. If I allow myself to be vulnerable and tell people that I sometimes struggle with feeling sad or anxious, they will reject me.	15	0—My vulnerability in relationships has actually helped others feel comfortable opening up to me.

If you compare the number of times your mind has made a negative social prediction to the number of times it has actually occurred, you might discover that your mind is often incorrect. How can you use this information to motivate yourself to take a social leap of faith when your worry, anxiety, and fear are begging you not to? A useful strategy can be to use an affirmation to remind yourself that your mind is not always right. Here are some examples of affirmations:

- I will not let the fears of my mind allow my social self-care to fall behind.
- This prediction won't cause me to stray away from my social conviction.

- I won't let my worries cause me to abandon my social self-care journey.
- My weather forecast says it's going to be dark and stormy. Never mind the weather, I'm taking this journey!

How to Handle Conflict in Relationships

Conflict is inevitable in all relationships. While we likely have a number of overlapping interests and perspectives with our partners, family, and friends, there are topics we simply do not agree on, and there will always be aspects of each other's personality that are irritating or off-putting. Contrary to what many of us are taught, disagreements and conflicts are not *bad*. In fact, if we handle them correctly they can help us feel more connected to one another. The determining factor of whether conflict has helpful or harmful effects is the quality of the communication that surrounds the conflict. Here are some tips for handling conflict in productive, healthy ways:

- **Listen.** Really make an effort to hear and understand the other person's perspective.
- **Express yourself.** Clearly and truthfully communicate your thoughts and feelings on the conflict. Use "I" statements to signal ownership of your thoughts, feelings, and behaviors.
- **Ask for what you need.** What do you need to resolve the issues and continue in this relationship?
- **Acknowledge the other person's feelings.** Try to see the other person's perspective and understand how they feel in the situation.
- **Be kind.** Be careful not to yell, insult, or call the other person names, or insult the other person's character.
- **Take a break if needed.** When things get too heated or it is clear that the conversation is not productive, take a break. Be sure to schedule a time to revisit and resolve the issue.
- **Avoid defensiveness.** Remember, it takes two to have an argument. Be willing to take responsibility for your role in the incident and apologize.

- **Come to a resolution and repair emotional harm.** Come to a clear understanding of what each person is willing to do differently to prevent a similar incident moving forward. Repair any emotional harm that was caused during the conflict to prevent resentment from setting in.

Your Commitment to Social Self-Care

Now it's time to make a commitment to live a life that's consistent with your social self-care vision. These steps will guide you toward shaping your relationships and social life around your values. Use your notebook to complete these steps.

1. Select an aspect of social self-care that you would like to focus on initially: social needs, engage, play, unwind, nurture, or grow.

2. Set a goal consistent with your values, and that's realistic given your schedule.

3. Cope ahead of time. Think about what could get in the way of pursuing your goal (for example, feeling unmotivated, unexpected illness, other responsibilities seem more pressing). What are some ways you can overcome these roadblocks?

4. Take action toward your goal.

5. Acknowledge your efforts. You're living out your values, and this is something to be celebrated!

6. In your notebook, take note of how the process of pursuing your goal went. What did you do that was effective and helped you achieve your goal? What barriers came up? Did you meet those barriers in an effective way? What might you do differently next time?

Once you've completed these steps, start again at step one. Pick a time interval that is most appropriate for you (weekly, biweekly, or monthly) and challenge yourself to engage in a behavior that supports your intention to prioritize social self-care. It could be as simple as playing with your dog after work or as elaborate as planning a gathering for a group of friends.

There are no limits here. Let your creativity run wild. The primary goal is to get in the habit of consistently doing something for yourself in the domain of social self-care. Remember to be flexible along the way. Life happens. Things don't always turn out as planned. Be kind to yourself when you get off track with your social self-care. You are doing the best you can. Commit to begin again.

Chapter Highlights

- Social self-care is nurturing your need for connection with other people. It involves taking care of existing relationships and friendships, creating new connections, and establishing boundaries in relationships with others.
- Your social self-care vision is a one-sentence declaration of the type of social self-care you desire. A vision helps you get clear about what you want your social self-care to look like, and it can serve as a guide for the decisions you will make in the future.
- When you are calm and in the moment, you are in a much better position to listen to what your body needs and wants, and you are poised to make choices that align with your social self-care vision.
- To stay healthy and connected, relationships need ongoing maintenance. This involves spending quality time together, engaging in activities that promote positive feelings toward one another, and expressing gratitude for appreciated actions and qualities.
- You can overcome challenges on your social self-care journey by acknowledging fears, anxieties, and worries for what they are; being accountable; and using effective communication during conflict.

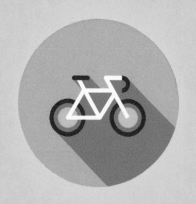

CHAPTER 3

Get Moving!
Physical Self-Care

Start with physical self-care if you want to:

- → Enhance your physical health
- → Improve your body image
- → Change your eating habits
- → Start exercising regularly
- → Sleep more soundly
- → Feel stronger, more confident, and healthier

Your Physical Needs

Physical self-care involves caring for your body in ways that sustain, revitalize, and strengthen it. When we do not take care of our bodies, we take the risk of becoming sick or not being able to move around as quickly and painlessly as we would like. Physical self-care gives our body the strength it needs to help us do the things we sometimes take for granted, like walk, run, swim, and dance. Physical self-care involves three components: physical movement, sleep and rest, and proper nutrition.

Physical movement carries a number of health benefits, including promoting improved brain functioning, enhanced sleep quality, and reduced risk of illness and disease. Doctors recommend that adults get two and a half to five hours per week of moderate-intensity exercise that gets our hearts pumping. Light bicycling, swimming, walking briskly, gardening, running, boxing, hiking, jogging, and playing a team sport, like basketball, are just a few exercises we can do for our cardiovascular health. In addition, we can keep ourselves physically strong by engaging in strength-training activities (such as lifting free weights or using weight machines), as well as bodyweight exercises (such as push-ups) and sports, like rock climbing.

We get the most benefit from physical activity when we do it consistently, and gradually challenge ourselves to reach the next level of intensity over time. Safety is also key! To prevent pain and possible injury, it's important to listen to your body and incorporate time for rest and recovery into your fitness routine.

Like exercise, sleep is extremely important for our day-to-day functioning. Adequate, regular sleep improves overall health and wellness by ensuring that we are functioning to the best of our ability—physically, mentally, and emotionally. To be at our best, doctors recommend that, as adults, we get seven to nine hours of sleep. I know many of us are functioning on far fewer hours than we need for some very legitimate reasons. At the same time, our goal should always be to consistently reach a minimum of seven hours. How well we sleep is just as important as the number of hours we spend in bed. Both quantity and quality are important.

Eating a healthy diet means getting proper nutrients and calories from the foods and beverages we eat. Poor eating habits and an inadequate diet have been linked to obesity and the development of preventable chronic conditions such as diabetes and cardiovascular disease. Foods and beverages that fuel our bodies the best include a range of vegetables, whole fruits, whole grains, low- or fat-free dairy, a variety of proteins, and water. For optimal health and wellness, calories from artificial sugars, saturated fats, and sodium should be limited, and calories from nutrient-rich foods and beverages should be maximized.

Physical self-care also includes the way we think and feel about our body. This is known as our body image. It includes what you say to yourself when you look in the mirror and how you perceive yourself with regard to physical attributes; body weight, shape, and height; and your sense of your ability to influence and change your body. People with a positive body image focus more on their physical abilities and feel comfortable and confident about their bodies no matter how the physical appearance of their bodies may change over time. A positive body image can support your physical self-care by helping you accept yourself and your body even though you may be taking steps to improve your physical health.

One way to improve your body image is to focus on a goal other than changing your body. Why? Well, from a very young age, family members and peers give us feedback about our body weight. Much of this feedback is laced with negative judgments and comparisons that leave us feeling ashamed. On top of that, we are bombarded with messages from the media about how our bodies should look. As you begin your journey toward enhanced physical self-care, I encourage you to change this narrative. Resist the urge to internalize negative messages, and focus instead on being grateful for the body you have and all it allows you to do.

Your Physical Self-Care Values

Here's an exercise to help you clarify your physical self-care values. Remember, values are like a life compass. They help guide your actions and motivate you to create meaningful habits. Get your notebook and answer the following questions.

- **Imagine that you live in a society where, as an incentive for physical self-care, each adult is given two hours a day to focus solely on their physical self-care each and every day.** You can work on your physical health in any environment you'd like and in any way you like. What would you do?
- **There are a variety of ways you can improve your physical self-care during your daily two-hour time block, but imagine that you could select only 10 activities from the following list.** (Don't worry: After 12 months have passed, you can switch it up.) In your notebook, write down the 10 activities you selected and rank them on a scale of 1 to 10, where 1 is the most important activity and 10 is the least important activity. Keep in mind that you can do more than one of your selected activities during the two-hour period. For example, you could take a one-hour nap, do 30 minutes of cardiovascular exercise, and eat a mindful meal. There are no right or wrong answers.
- **For each item on your list, evaluate why you chose that particular activity.** Why does it matter to you? In what way will that activity help enhance your physical self-care? Why is it important to you to enhance your physical self-care in this manner? For each activity you selected, complete the following sentence in your notebook: *This item is important to me because . . .*

Physical Self-Care Activities

- Cardiovascular fitness class (group or one-on-one)
- Coaching class or independent study on being kind and compassionate toward yourself when your actions are not in line with your physical self-care values
- Coaching class or independent study on developing a healthy body image
- Coaching class or independent study on how to eat in moderation and how to avoid overeating

- Coaching class or independent study on how to incorporate flexibility and balance into your eating habits and exercise routine
- Coaching class or independent study on how to unlearn unhelpful beliefs and attitudes about physical self-care
- Coaching class or independent study on improving sleep quantity and/or quality
- Coaching class or independent study on improving your health without shaming or punishing yourself
- Coaching class or independent study on maintaining a healthy physical self-care routine while traveling and during holidays and vacations
- Cooking class focused on a variety of healthy meals
- Cooking class focused on flavorful healthy meals
- Cooking class focused on quick healthy meals
- Cooking healthy meals on your own
- Dance class (type of dance is up to you!) (group or one-on-one)
- Eat a healthy meal together as a family
- Eat a mindful meal
- Engage in a healthy bedtime routine
- Engage in physical movement as a family, such as a family bike ride or walk
- Fitness class focused on improving flexibility and core strength (group or one-on-one)
- Martial arts class (group or one-on-one)
- Nap
- Nutrition class on changing unhealthy eating habits and improving your health without dieting
- Nutrition class on the main food groups
- Personal training session
- Practice making healthy choices at restaurants and social gatherings
- Strength-training class (group or one-on-one)
- Water exercise class or swimming
- Yoga class (group or one-on-one)

Obviously, we don't live in a society that requires us to engage in two hours of physical self-care daily. But imagining yourself in this scenario probably gave you a good idea of which type of physical activities you value. Knowing this can be the motivation you need to start taking action on your physical self-care.

Engage

One thing that makes physical self-care so hard is that there is no one-size-fits-all approach. Each person has their own optimal physical health, body size, and food preferences. There is no finish line. Physical self-care is something we will work toward until our time on Earth is up. Another challenge related to physical self-care is that our busy schedules do not seem to allow for choosing whole and healthy foods, adequate sleep, and consistent exercise.

Create a Physical Self-Care Schedule

Each week, perhaps on Sunday, before the workweek begins, spend some time planning how you'll do some physical self-care in the coming week. If you use a physical calendar, write in "physical self-care" on the days you selected. Pick the time, length, and frequency (throughout the week) that works best for you. If you use an electronic calendar, set an alarm to signal you that it is time for physical self-care. Protect this time as though it were an important appointment—because it is! Aside from an emergency, don't let anything get in the way of your scheduled physical self-care. If you must skip a session because something serious comes up, be sure to reschedule it.

During your physical self-care time, use the entire allotted time for your chosen activity. Minimize all distractions—for example, log out of your e-mail account and social media sites, silence your phone, close your door, make sure your kids are occupied or supervised, politely ask to be uninterrupted by those around you, and turn off the television.

Try Something New: Choose an Activity

Take another look at the list of physical self-care activities (see page 38). In your notebook, rate how willing you are to try each activity using a scale of 1 to 5, with 5 being very willing and 1 not being willing at all. From the activities you rate 5, pick just one activity to try. Answer the following questions in your notebook:

- Which activity did you choose?
- When will you try the new activity?
- How did it feel to do this activity?

Reflecting on how the activity went helps you determine if you want to try it again, modify it in some way to make it more enjoyable for you, or try a different high-ranking activity.

Making the Time: Create Openings for Exercise in Your Schedule

We're all busy and strapped for time, but I promise with a little creativity you *can* find time in your schedule for exercise. You can exercise for as long or short as your schedule allows; even short periods of exercise have been shown to produce health benefits.

The following steps can help you identify ways that you are willing to create an opening in your schedule and follow through on the activity. Remember to use your notebook to keep track of your intentions.

1. **Choose one behavior from either of these categories that you are willing to try this week:**

Making Time for Exercise with Creativity	Making Time for Exercise with Compromise
Start a lunchtime walking routine with colleagues.	Replace time on social media with exercise.
Engage in exercise with your pet, spouse, or kids (e.g., walk, run, dance challenge).	Replace time watching television with exercise.

Making Time for Exercise with Creativity	Making Time for Exercise with Compromise
Park at the far end of the parking lot.	Spend a portion of your lunch break engaged in physical activity.
Walk to destinations that are close by.	Get up 30 to 60 minutes earlier to allow time for exercise.
After leaving work, stop at the gym before you head home.	Instead of meeting a friend for dinner, invite them to take a walk or go for a run at a local park or take a class together.
When you watch television, exercise during commercials.	Instead of sleeping in pajamas, go to sleep in your work-out clothes as a reminder to get moving first thing in the morning.

2. **Notice any hesitancy that arises in the form of thoughts (for example, "I don't want to do that") or feelings such as anxiety.** This is normal. You are trying something outside of your comfort zone.

3. **State your intention and value.** Write the following in your notebook and say it out loud: *I am committed to (insert exercise activity) this week on (insert day of the week) from (insert start time) until (insert end time). I am willing to (restate exercise activity) because my physical self-care is important to me. My physical self-care is important to me because . . .*

   If you would like extra accountability, share your intention with a friend or family member and request that they check in with you after your planned activity. You can even post it on social media.

4. **Plan ahead.** Think through all that will need to happen in order for your intention to manifest. Will you need to pack gym clothes? Do you need to schedule an appointment? Do

you need to secure someone to pick up the kids from school? Do you need to initiate or renew your gym membership?

5. **Take action.** Remind yourself that you have only committed to try this once. Approach it as you would an experiment. Your job is to do the exercise to the best of your ability for the total allotted time, and observe your experience before, during, and after the exercise.

6. **Be fully present while engaging in the exercise.** A good way to stay present is to focus on your breath. Notice any thoughts, feelings, and bodily sensations that are present just before you begin the exercise, during the exercise, and after the exercise.

7. **Create the following chart in your notebook and fill it out as soon as you can after completing your activity.**

Experiment Reflections

	Before	During	After (Immediately and 30 minutes)
Thoughts			Immediate: 30 Minutes:
Feelings			Immediate: 30 Minutes:
Bodily Sensations			Immediate: 30 Minutes:

After you've taken these steps, spend a moment reflecting on your observations. Would you be willing to try this activity again? Why or why not? If yes, start over at step two and proceed through each step just like before. If no, start over at step one. The sooner you do this, the better chance you have of making it happen!

Eat

What we choose to put into our bodies affects everything from our mood to our cognitive functioning. Part of physical self-care is eating the foods that will nourish you and make you feel your best. These next exercises will guide you in developing eating habits to enhance your physical health.

Create a Healthy Meal Plan

Here's a step-by-step guide to assist you in creating a sustainable, long-term healthy meal plan:

1. In your notebook, devote half a page to each day of the week: Monday through Sunday. Beneath each day of the week, number your meals (typically, three to five meals per day).

2. Make a list of healthy and whole foods you would like to eat at each meal each day. Limit foods high in sugar and saturated fat. Make your meals colorful! Varied natural colors on your plate assures you that you are receiving a variety of nutrients from your food. Be sure to include the following (based on USDA guidelines for a 2,000-calorie diet) over the course of the day:

    Vegetables: 2 ½ cups

    Proteins: 5 ½ ounces

    Fruits: 2 cups

    Whole grains: 6 ounces

    Dairy: 3 cups

    Oils/healthy fats: 27 grams

3. Decide whether you prefer to cook daily, every other day, or once weekly. Create a shopping list from the foods you listed, keeping in mind the frequency you will be cooking, and shop accordingly. See the tips for healthy grocery shopping to follow.

4. At the end of the week, evaluate how your plan is working. Make adjustments as needed.

Here are some tips to maximize your chances of sticking with your plan: If you intend to cook daily, make sure that all food items are properly thawed and ready to be cooked each day. If you choose to prepare meals ahead of time, start small and see how it goes. When you're ready, you can advance to preparing precooked meals that you can just grab, go, and reheat during your busy week. Again, it's best to start small. Slow cookers can be your best friend when your schedule is busy and you need a full nutritious meal without a sink full of dirty dishes. The Internet is full of handy slow-cooker recipes.

Tips for Healthy Grocery Shopping

These guidelines can help guide you in making decisions that support your physical self-care during your next trip to the grocery store.

- Make a grocery list based on meals and healthy snacks you plan to eat over the next week and stick to it.
- Avoid grocery shopping when you're hungry or rushed. Hunger makes you more likely to choose foods that are highly processed (because you want to eat *now*). Set aside enough time to grocery shop so that you can properly read labels and pick the freshest meats and produce.
- Opt for whole foods over processed meals.
- The more colorful your cart the better.
- Frozen veggies are a healthy option and can help you save on cooking time during the week. Choose the ones with no seasoning or sauce.

- When purchasing canned goods, choose options without added salt or juice.
- Avoid aisles with processed foods and foods high in sugar. If you don't see them, you won't buy them! Stick with the aisles where you'll find fresh fruits, vegetables, whole grains, dairy, and meat.

"EATING IS AN EXPERIENCE, NOT A MEANS TO AN END."
—DR. ROBYN L. GOBIN

EATING MINDFULLY MEANS...

SLOWING DOWN

Eat at a leisurely pace. Notice how your body feels before, during, and after eating.

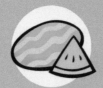

PAYING ATTENTION

Observe what you eat, why you eat, and how you eat. Notice the influence of emotions, thoughts, and surroundings on your eating patterns.

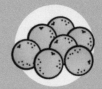

FULLY ENGAGING

Give the meal your full attention. Minimize distractions such as reading, talking, watching TV, and browsing social media.

SENSING

Engage in a sense of sight, touch, smell, sound, and taste while eating. Taste and savor your food.

BEING CURIOUS

Approach each meal with an open mind. Be willing to learn something new about your food likes and dislikes.

BEING KIND

Be gentle, patient, and nurturing towards your body and your struggles with food.

WWW.ROBYNGOBIN.COM

- Check ingredients lists. The fewer ingredients the better. This likely means that the food has few additives and is not overly processed.

Mindful Eating

When it comes to eating, many of us approach meals like we're in a competition to see who can eat the most food in the fastest amount of time. We eat fast and furiously only to get to the end of a meal and find ourselves feeling overly stuffed and sluggish. It's a shame that we have developed this type of a relationship with food because eating has so much pleasure to offer—if only we would slow down enough to pay attention.

Mindful eating is a way to offer yourself physical self-care. Mindful eating means paying attention to what you are eating while you are eating. It's a pathway to developing a healthier relationship with food. Rather than viewing food as problematic or a "quick fix" for soothing unwanted emotions, you can view food as a source of fuel for your body and, in doing so, free yourself from fears, obsessions, and addictions that surround food in our culture. Mindful eating invites you to release fear-based food aversions (for example, "I don't like vegetables") and habits, and instead let your eating behaviors be guided by *your own* experience in the here and now. Try eating one meal a day mindfully.

Sleep

Although we've all heard the benefits of a good night's rest, sleep is highly underrated in our society—so much so that we wear exhaustion and sleep deprivation like badges of honor to be admired. I've even heard people joke, "Sleep is overrated. I'll sleep when I'm dead!" We've learned to function on way less than the recommended seven to nine hours. Instead, we rely on caffeine and willpower to get us through. Because we can *technically* function this way, we come to adopt a perpetual state of being sleep deprived as the norm.

Scientific evidence on the negative effects of not getting enough good-quality sleep is clear: Sleep deprivation is linked to physical and mental health problems, impaired brain functioning and decision-making, memory difficulties, injuries, reduced productivity, and a greater risk of accidental death.

The remedy for chronic sleep deprivation involves realizing and honoring our human limits. Sleep is a basic physical need. Fulfilling this need requires us to establish priorities, limit the responsibilities we take on, and get comfortable with leaving items undone on our to-do lists. This is no easy feat in a world that rewards us for pushing ourselves beyond our limits, but it's possible. When we're fully rested, we can function better during the day, make better decisions, be more productive, and experience more pleasure in life. The following exercises will help you improve physical self-care in the area of sleep.

Start a Healthy Bedtime Routine

How do you signal to your body that it is time for sleep? Do you lie in bed and watch TV or YouTube? Do you catch up on all the latest news on social media? Or do you turn off all the lights and lie there ruminating about all the things that went wrong during the day?

If you said yes to any of the above, you could benefit from establishing a bedtime routine. This is a set of behaviors you do before bedtime to signal to your brain that it is time for sleep. The following steps provide a foundation for setting yourself up for high-quality sleep:

1. **Stay active and busy throughout your day.** When it is time for bed, you will be tired and ready to fall asleep.

2. **Set a consistent bedtime.** Choose a time when you will be tired enough to want to go to bed but also one that will allow for a minimum of seven hours of sleep.

3. **Avoid watching TV, scrolling through social media, and working in bed.** This helps to signal to your body that the bed is for sleep and sleep only.

4. **Signal to your body that it's bedtime by doing one or more of the following:**

  - Change into your sleep clothes.

  - Brush your teeth.

  - Take a bath or shower.

  - Drink non-caffeinated tea.

  - Turn off all screens, including television, smartphones, computers, and laptops.

  - Listen to a guided sleep meditation or bedtime story for adults. Several options are available online via YouTube or Mindfulness Meditation mobile applications, such as Calm, Headspace, or Insight Timer.

  - Engage in a mindful breathing exercise focused on paying attention to the physical sensations of breathing.

  - Turn off the lights and eliminate any distracting noises.

5. **Get comfortable.** Invest in a comfortable mattress, pillows, and sheets. Set a temperature that is optimal for you when you sleep. Dress in a manner that will keep you comfortable throughout the night.

6. **Minimize the amount of time you spend awake in bed.** If you have trouble falling asleep within the first 10 to 15 minutes of getting into bed, get out of bed and try one of these two strategies:

  If you can't stop thinking about what you have to do tomorrow, write a to-do list. Try to "leave it all on the paper."

  Turn on a low reading light, and read something you find boring. If all else fails, grab a dictionary. No reading or playing on your phone. Once you feel yourself getting sleepy, get back in bed. Repeat if you are still unable to fall asleep.

When you take time to create the right conditions for a restful night's sleep, you will be more likely to sleep well, which will benefit every other aspect of your physical self-care efforts.

Reward Yourself

To enhance the quality of your sleep and reward yourself for making your sleep routine a priority, consider one or more of the following:

- Buy a set of nice sheets.
- Purchase a background noise machine that makes relaxing sounds such as waterfalls, rain, or wind blowing.
- Gift yourself a new pair of PJs.
- Try a new bodywash or shampoo with a soothing scent.
- Drink a cup of herbal tea.

Move

The key to enhancing your physical activity is to start small. There are a range of possibilities for becoming more active. Maybe you can't make it to the gym four times a week. That is okay. As the saying goes, "The race is not won to the swift but him who endureth till the end." The goal is to find a level of physical activity that is challenging enough to get you in shape, but not so punishing that you won't be able to sustain it.

What's most important is that you move more, no matter your current lifestyle or physical limitations. You can gradually increase your "more" as life circumstances allow. This is not about achieving some ideal weight or "perfect" body; rather, the goal is to continue moving closer to the ideals you outlined in the physical self-care values exercise (see page 38). Remember, your reason for getting healthier is to maximize what your body can do for you. A question you can ask yourself to keep you connected to this mind-set is: "What will I be able to do with a healthier body?" Use the answer as your motivation to get moving!

Add Informal Physical Activity to Your Day

You don't have to go to the gym or join a team sport to get your blood pumping. You can simply do the things you already do in a more active way. Here are some ideas to get you going:

- **Take the stairs.** Whenever you have to choose between an elevator, escalator, or stairs, always choose stairs. Climbing the stairs is a surefire way to get your heart pumping!
- **Park in the back.** Rather than circling the parking lot trying to find the perfect spot near the front of your destination, park further away to increase your step count.
- **Don't take a "lazy load."** When I was growing up, this was one of my mother's favorite sayings whenever she'd come home with a trunk full of groceries and I would try to take all 20 bags in at once. Instead of trying to bring all of your grocery bags inside in one trip, split it up into several trips. Same goes for the laundry. After you finish the laundry, let it take you several trips to put the clean linens and clothing in their designated spaces. You're moving more just by getting your chores done.
- **Keep your home tidy.** Yep, that's right. Get in the habit of vacuuming, cleaning windows, mopping, scrubbing the bathroom, and dusting regularly to keep you active.
- **Beautify your lawn.** Yard work is a terrific way to fit in physical activity.
- **Use public transportation.** When you need to run an errand, go to work, or head to an appointment, consider taking the bus or train. You'll likely need to walk from the bus or train to get to your final destination, which is a win for your physical self-care.
- **Try walking meetings.** Instead of seated meetings, discuss your agenda items while taking a walk. When I was in graduate school, my mentor had regular meetings with all of her mentees that became fondly known as "walk and talks."
- **Take evening walks.** How do you usually unwind or connect with family members after dinner? Try creating a new routine of evening walks with loved ones. It's a great way to fit in physical activity while catching up on the highlights of everyone's day.

And, as you're increasing your physical activity, be sure to drink more water. Increased water intake helps make your body healthier by flushing out unnecessary toxins.

Create Community Activities That Get People Moving

Many of us are members of groups in our communities, whether it be at work, school, or our place of worship. A fun way to get moving is to incorporate group-based physical activity into groups you already belong to. In addition to being able to spend quality time with people you like, you have built-in accountability that can help motivate you to stay committed to your physical self-care.

Is it possible for you to get together with members of your congregation or colleagues and do something active together on weekends? Would it be possible to organize a Saturday morning walk in your neighborhood or at a local school or park? If you're a business owner, how could you structure the work environment in a way that promotes physical activity? Would you be willing to invest in a company-sponsored on-site gym or allow employees to leave 30 minutes early one day a week as an investment in their physical self-care?

There are a lot of possible ways to promote group physical activities. Grab your notebook and answer these questions to get your creative juices flowing.

- In what ways can you make it easier to be physically active with family, colleagues, peers, teammates, and congregation members in your community?
- What activity will you focus on first? Why?
- What is one action you can take now to support your goal of creating a healthier family, work, school, or faith community?

With your answers in hand, take that one action as soon as you can to make this part of your physical self-care plan a reality.

Grow

Two of the biggest barriers to prioritizing your physical self-care are unrealistic expectations and time management. When we learn how to set realistic expectations and manage our time more effectively, we can experience growth in the area of physical self-care.

Set Realistic Expectations

If you start this process with unrealistic expectations, it could prevent you from sticking with your physical self-care goals: They can lead to reduced motivation and make you more likely to abandon your physical self-care routine when you don't see the results you expected. Here are a few signs that may indicate you have unrealistic expectations for your physical self-care routine:

- Expecting perfection.
- Expecting fast results.
- Being overly critical or harsh with yourself when you lapse into old habits (for example, calling yourself names or punishing yourself).
- Using the words "should" or "always" when referring to yourself.
- Having strict, inflexible rules for yourself around certain types of food, physical activities, or body size.
- Your primary goal for physical self-care is to control your body—its size, shape, etc.

One way to help you set more realistic expectations is to change what you focus on in your physical self-care journey. Instead of focusing on achieving a specific weight or body type, focus on how you feel. Do you feel stronger? Healthier? Happier? Proud? Committed? Consistent? Focus on how your body feels and what your body can do for you.

Approach your physical self-care with curiosity. View it as an opportunity to learn new things about yourself and grow. What character traits are you building by prioritizing your physical self-care? Focus more on your wins than on your losses and slipups. View your slipups as learning opportunities. What did you learn that you can use to help you make a different choice in the future? When you focus on these things, your expectations become more realistic.

Manage Time Effectively

Here's the deal with time: We all have the same 24 hours in each day. Within that, we make time for necessities like sleeping and eating, and we also make time for the things that matter most to us. I know it can feel like all the responsibilities and people in your life are making demands on your time to the point that there's essentially no time left for physical self-care. Can I let you in on a little secret? *You* get to choose how you spend your time. When you learn to manage your time more effectively, you can create more time for physical self-care. Here are some strategies for managing your time more effectively:

- **Plan.** To make the best use of the 24 hours you have every day, it is essential to plan out your day. It can be useful to write or type out your schedule on a physical or electronic calendar to keep you on task throughout the day.
- **Set priorities.** When planning your day, prioritize your physical self-care first. This means committing to include physical self-care somewhere in your schedule. Adopt the mind-set that says, "My physical self-care is nonnegotiable." Then, prioritize the tasks you want to complete each day. What is most important to get done each day? What activities will have the highest payoff as it relates to your overall goals in this area of your life?
- **Be realistic.** Being realistic involves accurately predicting how much time it will take to accomplish a given task. Do you tend to overestimate or underestimate how long it will take you to do tasks? If so, set a timer to give you an accurate sense of how much time you are spending on specific activities so that you can build in the accurate amount of time when planning out your schedule. You might also find that you are dedicating too much (or too little) time to certain tasks. If this is the case, consider reallocating your time.
- **Commit cautiously.** When you are given the choice to take on new opportunities, responsibilities, or roles, don't say yes right away. Take the time to consider whether you truly have time for the new

task given your physical self-care and overall self-care goals and whether the task aligns with your values. If not, consider saying no.

- **Minimize distractions at work.** Offer your best work by devoting your undivided attention to it. Close out of your e-mails, put away your phone, appear "away" on your company instant-messaging service, close your door, and get to work. This will give you more time for your physical self-care routine later.

- **Take breaks.** This is your time to stretch, take a walk, check e-mail, eat, or scroll through social media. Research has shown that we are most effective when we work in predetermined chunks of time. Taking breaks helps ensure that you have the appropriate focus, energy, and attention to sustain you. Breaks are most effective when you do things that you can easily transition out of. Be sure to set a timer so that your break doesn't run longer than you intended it to.

- **Minimize procrastination.** When you have things to do, resist the urge to wait until the last possible minute to get them done. The sooner you do what needs to be done, the sooner you can do pleasurable things without the weight of guilt or anxiety from those items looming on your to-do list.

- **Do one thing at a time.** Our culture has bamboozled us into thinking we are most efficient when we multitask. However, research has shown that we are actually less efficient when we do more than one task at a time. It is less efficient because your brain needs to switch back and forth between tasks. Rather than bouncing back and forth between tasks, set a predetermined amount of time for each task and stick to it.

- **Delegate.** To make the most of your time, you will need to learn how to delegate tasks to others with the skill and ability to complete the task. It's a great way to build your leadership skills while making sure that your physical self-care needs are met. WARNING: This will require you to let go of tendencies toward perfectionism. Be willing to allow things to get done even if they are not done perfectly or the way you would have done them. Think through your daily tasks and consider if there are things you can delegate to family members, friends, colleagues, or kids. If your finances allow, can you pay someone to clean your home or babysit while you engage in physical self-care?

- **Embrace being versus doing.** This is another way of saying, "Be okay with doing nothing." Our society fosters an addiction to busyness that makes us feel like we're not being productive if we're not doing *something*. This is a lie. Learn to be okay with slowing down and having blocks of spare time in your schedule. When you have free time, think of it as an opportunity to practice physical self-care (or any other domain of self-care).

Your Commitment to Physical Self-Care

Take a moment to revisit "Your Physical Self-Care Values" (see page 37). You identified 10 aspects of physical self-care and described why each was most important to you. Use this to guide you as you make decisions about physical self-care moving forward. It can be helpful to choose one of the 10 aspects to focus on each week. With this one aspect of physical self-care in mind, ask yourself the following question at the end of each day: "Is this (food, physical activity, or sleep) choice in the service of my physical self-care?"

If the answer is no, what is one action you can commit to for tomorrow that is consistent with your values with respect to physical self-care? Complete this statement in your notebook: *The one action I commit to taking tomorrow that is consistent with my physical self-care is: (fill in activity). I will take this action because . . .*

Chapter Highlights

- Physical self-care has three main components: physical movement, sleep and rest, and proper nutrition.
- A positive body image can support your physical self-care by helping you accept yourself and your body, even while working to improve your physical health.
- Mindful eating provides an avenue for offering yourself physical self-care. Mindful eating involves paying attention to what you are eating and how you are eating while you are eating. It is a pathway to developing a healthier relationship with food.
- Even short periods of exercise have been shown to produce health benefits.
- Sleep is a basic human need. Fulfilling this need requires establishing priorities, limiting the responsibilities you take on, and getting comfortable with leaving items undone on your to-do list.
- When you learn to set realistic expectations and manage your time more effectively, you can experience growth and expansion in the area of physical self-care.

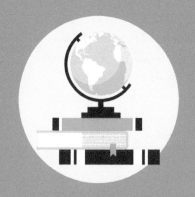

CHAPTER 4

The Life of the Mind
Intellectual Self-Care

START HERE IF

Start with intellectual self-care if you want to:

→ Stimulate your mind
→ Expand your knowledge
→ Widen your perspective
→ Deepen your creativity
→ Exercise your curiosity

Your Intellectual Needs

The brain is one of the most underrated parts of the body. It's *always* working, even when we are unaware that it's at work. Our brain helps us judge and evaluate situations, make plans, solve complex problems, and remember the past. For such a small part of our body (only about three pounds!), it has massive responsibility. Because the brain operates so effortlessly, it can be easy to forget just how vulnerable it is to diminished performance over the course of our lives. We all know that physical exercise and movement are necessary for the body to stay strong and healthy. Well, the same is true for our brains.

To help your brain function to the best of its ability for as long as possible, you need to exercise it. Intellectual self-care is exercise for your brain; it's doing things that keep your brain sharp. It is a lifelong commitment to learning new things that includes opening yourself up to unfamiliar experiences, exercising your creativity, and challenging your brain to solve problems and embrace knowledge. When you exercise your brain, it helps you function better across the board. I've seen intellectual self-care work wonders in my own life, as well as in the lives of my clients.

You might be thinking, "I'm okay with learning new things, but I'm not into reading technical books or playing mind-training games." The good news is that learning doesn't have to be boring, and it does not need to look like it did when you were in school. You don't have to read long books or listen to someone lecturing you. There are plenty of ways to stimulate your brain without feeling like you are going to die of boredom or dredging up old painful memories of feeling dumb in chemistry class. Reading a book, magazine, or blog for pleasure; listening to an informational podcast or an audiobook; playing cards; solving crosswords; playing Wordscapes or other games on your smartphone; visiting a museum; or engaging in healthy debate on a topic you're passionate about—all these fun activities also exercise your brain.

What Do You Want Your Brain to Do for You?

To take care of our brains, we need a clear understanding of all that our brains do for us. The following is a list of activities your brain makes possible for you:

Compete	Perceive (ability to use
Contemplate	five senses)
Cooperate	Plan
Create	Pray
Decide	Process new information
Experience and express	Read
emotions	Remember
Focus/pay attention	Respond to my
Judge	environment
Label (experiences and	Speak/communicate
emotions)	Study
Meditate	Think
Move (walk, run, play, etc.)	Understand
Observe	Use my intuition

In your notebook, jot down the top three brain activities that are most important to you. For each item, respond to these three questions:

1. **"What does this brain function allow me to do that matters to me?"** Here are two examples:

    Creating helps me come up with new ways of organizing my home.

    Perception helps me to be able to smell.

2. **"Why is that important to me?"** Here are two examples:

    Creating new ways of organizing my home is important to me because it helps me maintain structure and feel in control of my life.

    It is important for me to be able to smell because I enjoy scented candles.

3. **"What am I doing to nurture this brain function so that it stays strong?"** If nothing, what can you start doing to nurture this brain function? Here are two examples:

> To help my brain think to the best of its ability, I am willing to start listening to a podcast that focuses on the topics of organization and productivity.

> To help enhance my perception, I am willing to practice mindfulness so that I can deepen my ability to savor the candle scents I enjoy.

The list of what our brain does for us is virtually endless, and the same is true for the ways we can help support it so that it functions at its best. Start with one simple act today to help your brain do what you need and want it to do.

Engage

If you're like most people, it's probably been a while since you've thought about all the things your brain does for you, much less considered exercising your brain. This section shows you why prioritizing intellectual self-care is important, and how to start doing it. Simply put, intellectual self-care keeps us sharp and growing. One of the easiest ways to ward off boredom or a sense of feeling stuck is to keep challenging yourself to learn and grow.

Where to Start: Learn More About an Interesting Topic

We all find certain things interesting. Learning more about the topics you already enjoy can be a great place to start when you want to stimulate your brain. Grab your notebook and make a list of all the topics, activities, sports, places, people, and even animals you find interesting—things you're curious about, that excite you, and really hold your attention.

Once you have this list, think about ways to learn more about the stuff that interests you. For instance, one of my favorite sports to watch is boxing. I admire the amount of technique and skill it takes to have the stamina to last 12 rounds in the ring, and I love the fact that, at any moment, one move can change the whole fight. The excitement of it all is thrilling to me! One way I've used my joy for boxing to contribute to my intellectual self-care is by getting to know specific boxers. I treat it like a fun history lesson, and search for articles about the man or woman behind the gloves. In the process of doing this research I'm gaining new knowledge, which helps me feel more connected to the sport. After I learn something new about a particular boxer, I share the information with my husband. By recalling what I learned and sharing this information, I'm exercising my memory.

One of my colleagues enjoys keeping track of current events in the lives of her favorite celebrities. How about you? Can you think of a topic you'd enjoy reading about online or in a magazine?

Try Something New: Learn a Language

Learning a new language is an excellent way to feed your brain and keep it in shape. It helps keep your mind sharp by demanding that it translate information that you read or heard from your native language to the language you are learning. At the same time, learning a new language sharpens your communication skills and opens up the possibilities for you to create new relationships with people who speak the language you are learning.

There are so many cool ways to learn a new language these days. There are books, apps, study abroad programs, and personal language coaches. *And* there are tons of languages to learn. Take a moment to consider what language you might be interested in learning. Take one step in that direction by downloading a language learning app—such as Duolingo, Memrise, or Busuu—on your phone and spending some time exploring the app.

Making the Time: Find "Free Moments" for Intellectual Stimulation

What if I told you that creating time for intellectual stimulation doesn't necessarily require you to carve out time in your schedule? It can be as simple as repurposing the time you already have. We all have "free moments" that sneak by each day without our even recognizing it. For example, moments tick by while we are waiting for appointments, classes, or meetings to begin; while commuting to and from work; while standing in line or sitting on hold; while commercials are playing; and so on. This doesn't even include the time we spend checking our phones and scrolling through social media.

Imagine if you decided to repurpose just a fraction of these "free moments" on intellectual self-care. Here are a few ideas for doing just that:

- Listen to an audiobook or podcast.
- Read a newspaper, book, or blog.
- Play a game on your smartphone that requires you to think, solve a problem, or get creative. Flow Free, UNO, Wheel of Fortune, Solitaire, and Draw It are just a few of the game apps you can download.
- Engage with a language learning app.
- Nurture your creativity by coming up with an invention that would make your life easier.

Taking just a few moments for these mind-stimulating activities when you would otherwise be wasting time waiting for something to happen goes a long way in nurturing your intellectual self-care.

Discover

Sometimes it can be hard to know (or remember!) what truly interests us. Life has a way of pulling us toward doing the things that are necessary, like paying bills and keeping our household running (in other words, *adulting*) to the extent that we can forget we also need to be engaging our mind in meaningful ways. If we give ourselves the chance to wake up out of the fog of autopilot, we might realize that we don't even know what topics or hobbies we find intriguing. This "Get to Know Your Interests" activity can lay the foundation for discovering what appeals to you most and which interests and pastimes are going to feed your brain the nourishment it needs.

Get to Know Your Interests

One way to learn more about topics that excite you is to pay close attention to how you feel when you're engaging in different activities to try to stimulate your mind. To get you started, here's a list of topics to choose from, or come up with your own:

Climate	Movies
Culture	Music
Geography	Politics
History	Public health
Law	Science
Math	Technology
Medicine	Visual/performing arts
Mental health	Women's issues/history

Now, grab your notebook and create a grid like the one that follows. I've included an example for you to follow. For the next week, commit to "trying on" a topic or activity to see how much it interests and excites you on a scale of 0 to 10, where 0 is not at all interested or excited and 10 is extremely interested or excited.

To explore the new topic, come up with an activity that exposes you to it. Possible activities include reading about the topic, listening to a podcast on the topic, talking to someone whose work revolves around that topic, or researching the topic on the Internet. Pay attention to how you feel when you are engaging in the activity. Notice whether you get absorbed in it and are eager to learn more or if you quickly lose interest. Pay attention to the types of thoughts and feelings you have while you are "trying on" the topic. The more excited and interested you feel, the more likely this is a topic you enjoy and may want to explore at a deeper level to nourish your mind.

Getting to Know Myself Log

Topic	Activity	Interest (0–10)	Excitement (0–10)
Example: History	Visit a Local Museum	6	8

Excite

Maybe it's been years since you've taken the time to think about the topics and ideas that really excite you. Make today the day you give yourself permission to reconnect with your intellectual side and really discover what topics make you feel eager to learn more. The following activity can help you remember what ideas and intellectual pursuits are exciting to you.

Connect with Your Inner Child

Remembering back to when you were a child is one way to help you rediscover topics that interest you. Try it now: Close your eyes. Think back to your childhood and answer these questions:

- When you were little, what did you want to be when you grew up?
- When you were in school, what classes were you enthusiastic about?
- What did you hunger to learn more about?

Answering these questions can give you a starting point by reconnecting you with the feeling of what it is like to be fully captivated, excited, and intrigued by a specific topic. Really allow yourself to travel back in time and connect with how you felt when you were a child—full of possibility, untainted by the mental roadblocks and real-life limitations that come with time and age. Grab your notebook and write down the topics that come to mind.

Reward Yourself

To reward yourself for nurturing your intellectual self-care, take a trip to your local bookstore or browse the book section of your favorite online retailer. Give yourself ample time to browse around and check out different genres. Buy any book that strikes your fancy. It doesn't have to be serious or intellectual—just anything that involves your mind. It could be a book of jokes or a paperback romance. Don't forget to actually take the time to read your new book for pleasure and to stimulate your mind.

Learn

Now that you have a better idea of the types of topics that excite you, it's time to start learning more about them. There are a variety of ways to learn—it's not all reading books and taking notes! You can acquire new knowledge by listening to experts on the radio or podcasts, doing something new with your hands, watching YouTube videos, and doing exercises that test the new knowledge you're gaining along the way.

Keep in mind that to really master a new skill or topic, you should practice it and engage with it consistently. Aim for daily or weekly contact to ensure the new knowledge really sinks in. For instance, if you want to learn the skill of driving, it is best to practice a few times a week to begin to master the skill. If you drive one day for one hour and don't drive again for several weeks, that increases the chances you will lose the new skills you acquired during your first lesson. Since you've picked topics that you find interesting or are otherwise motivated to pursue, working them into your weekly schedule should be fun.

Discover Your Learning Style

When you want to learn something new, it's important to know how you learn best. Researchers have identified four learning dimensions. Everyone falls somewhere along each of these four axes. Read the following descriptions and make a mental note of where you fall on each of the four dimensions.

- **Visual vs. Verbal.** This dimension has to do with how you prefer information to be presented to you. People who learn best by seeing (e.g., watching demonstrations or videos) are called *visual learners.* They learn best when they see images, charts, illustrations, and timelines. Verbal learners learn best by hearing. They learn best when new topics are described in plain language—either written or verbal—and they can talk through and summarize new knowledge they have gained in their own words.
- **Sensing vs. Intuitive.** This dimension has to do with how you tend to take in information. Sensing learners prefer for information to be concrete and practical. They learn best with facts, data, and repetition. Intuitive learners are more abstract in the way they think. They prefer to discover new concepts, and they like to understand the theory behind facts.
- **Active vs. Reflective.** This dimension has to do with how you process or understand new information. People who learn best by experimenting and doing something "hands on" with new information are called *active learners.* They learn best when they can see the "material come to life" and physically touch, create, or build things based on what they're learning. Reflective learners prefer to take their time and think things through before trying them out. While active learners enjoy group work, reflective learners prefer working alone.
- **Sequential vs. Global.** This dimension has to do with how you prefer to organize information you are learning. Sequential learners prefer to learn in small steps where concepts gradually build on one another in a linear, logical fashion. Global learners like to look at the "big picture" and take larger leaps in putting information together.

Once you know your personal learning style, you'll be able to figure out the best way to acquire new knowledge and the kind of setting in which you learn best. For example, if you are a visual learner, turn to videos and illustrated texts or go to live demonstrations. If you are a verbal learner, put your earbuds in and soak up the information. If you learn more by doing, get your hands to work.

Be SMART

To set yourself up for success when learning something new, it's best to set SMART goals. SMART is an acronym for Specific, Measurable, Achievable, Relevant, and Time Bound. Let's take a closer look at what that means and how it can help you set useful goals.

- **Specific (what?)** A specific goal states exactly what you are aiming to accomplish.
- **Measurable (how?)** A measurable goal says how you will accomplish what you want.
- **Achievable (realistic and doable)** An achievable goal is one that you can actually accomplish in a set period of time. It takes into account how long it takes to achieve the goal and how much time you have to put into working toward that goal.
- **Relevant (related to the goal)** A relevant goal is one that meets your specific needs in a given domain—in this case, intellectual self-care.
- **Time bound (when?)** A time-bound goal has a clear beginning and ending. It provides a deadline of when you expect to achieve your goal.

Let's look at an example: Say that my goal is to learn Italian. A SMART way to phrase this goal is: *My goal is to download the Babbel app and practice Italian for 10 minutes three times a week for the next month.* This goal is specific, because I spell out exactly what I plan to do. By saying that I will practice 10 minutes three times a week, the goal is measurable. It is relevant to my overall goal of nurturing my intellectual self-care. Finally, the goal is time bound because I said I would do this for a month.

Take out your notebook and practice writing a SMART goal for learning a skill or discovering more about a topic you enjoy.

Grow

When we nourish our intellectual self-care by learning a new skill, trying something that doesn't come easy to us, or even acquiring new knowledge by engaging in a new activity, we're bound to make mistakes. As adults, this early stage of the learning process can be challenging, even embarrassing, because we're accustomed to mostly doing tasks we've already mastered. Essentially, when we learn something new, we have to own that fact that we don't know something and humble ourselves enough to be taught by someone who *does* know. This can be difficult, because we all like to feel competent. Another challenge is *persistence*: When we try something for the first time and aren't good at it, it can be tough to convince ourselves to try it again. It can feel like a losing battle.

I'll give you an example from my own life. I learned how to swim at the age of 33. Let me tell you, that first lesson was rough! The instructor started me off by having me make my way around the edge of the pool, holding the wall, and bob up and down to get comfortable holding my breath under water. It wasn't super comfortable, but it was doable. But then she asked me to float in the water on my stomach, away from the safety of the wall. I tried it twice, but my fear of drowning cemented my feet to the bottom of the pool, and I could not, for the life of me, get both of my feet to come off the floor of the pool. Feeling embarrassed and defeated, I stood in the middle of the lap pool next to my swim instructor and started bawling. She was very reassuring, and I managed to pull myself together to wrap up my first lesson. A few days later, when it was time for my second lesson, I really, really wanted to cancel. But because I'm a stickler for finishing things I start, I went back for the second lesson, and the third, and the fourth.

In all, I ended up having more than 15 swim lessons. Although I wouldn't describe swimming as my number one go-to recreational activity, I can now say that I know the basics of swimming. For me, that is a *huge* feat! The reason I now know how to swim is because, despite feeling incompetent, self-conscious, and afraid, I was persistent. Lesson after lesson, no matter how much I didn't want to be there, I showed up, and no matter how things went, I went back for the next practice session. I credit my ability to show up to two mind-sets that will be an important part of integrating your new self-care practices: beginner's mind and the growth mind-set.

Beginner's Mind

"Beginner's mind" is a phrase that's used to describe a state of mind that helps you notice what is new and exciting, even in a familiar experience. It's the idea that no matter how many times you have experienced an activity, person, place, or thing, each new time you encounter it, it is new. It involves the ability to approach something familiar as if it were the first time you've ever encountered it—releasing all judgments, expectations, and predictions about how it will turn out.

Take, for example, Mondays. Mondays are challenging for many adults. We're coming off of the fun and relaxation of the weekend, and the reality of a new workweek is setting in. We have all types of preconceived notions about how the day will go, often just hoping that we can get by until quitting time. But what if, instead of projecting all our negative expectations onto each new Monday, we approached it as if it were the first Monday we've ever had? How would that mind-set change our attitude and perspective? I was able to show up to swim lessons each week not expecting it to be a total disaster because I let go of what happened at the previous lesson and approached the new lesson with fresh eyes. Beginner's mind transformed the activity for me. My mind wasn't clouded by prejudgments of how the lesson would unfold. I was open to the possibilities of what could happen.

Follow these five steps to practice beginner's mind while nurturing intellectual self-care through learning:

1. Start by noticing all the judgments, memories, and expectations you have.

2. See if it is possible to let go of them, letting them become like background noise.

3. Now turn your attention to the activity you are doing.

4. Fully participate in the experience by paying attention to what you are doing and not letting distractions take you away from the experience.

5. Focus on every aspect of what you are learning.

When you approach an activity with a beginner's mind using these steps, you are opening yourself up to a world of new possibilities and experiences.

The Growth Mind-set

A growth mind-set supports your intellectual self-care by helping you stay open to challenging yourself mentally. When you have a growth mind-set, you believe you can grow and improve your abilities with consistent effort. What's more, you believe that you *should* be constantly learning and growing—that it's an essential part of life. From the perspective of a growth mind-set, setbacks and even failures are viewed as opportunities to learn and improve. When you adopt a growth mind-set, you're more focused on the process of learning than on getting to an outcome.

A growth mind-set is more about enjoying the journey than focusing on the destination. In contrast, a *fixed* mind-set is the exact opposite—and it can be a roadblock to growth. It assumes either you are good at something or you're not. People with a fixed mind-set prefer not to take risks or do things that expose them to the possibility of failure.

Take a look at the characteristics described in the following chart. Does the right or left side describe you most? If you discover that you have more of a fixed mind-set, I have good news for you: You can develop more of a growth mind-set. All it takes is shifting your perspective to focus on how much you are learning and growing rather than on the end result.

Fixed Mind-set	Growth Mind-set
Either you are naturally good at something or you are not.	Your performance can be improved with consistency and effort.
Failure is bad.	Failure is a chance to learn.
Feedback is bad.	Feedback helps me improve.
Prefer easy tasks that require minimal effort.	Prefer challenging tasks that require effort.
Give up easily in the face of barriers.	Persist in the face of barriers.
Focus on the end goal.	Focus on the journey.
Avoid risks.	Take risks.

Your Commitment to Intellectual Self-Care

Look back at the "What Do You Want Your Brain to Do for You?" exercise (see page 61). Grab your notebook and write down one thing you are willing to do in the next week to support your brain in doing the things you want it to do for you.

Now, imagine what barriers might come up as you are preparing to take this action. It could be an internal battle like not being in the mood or having a headache, or it could be an external barrier like you have an older car and you had plans to go to the museum, but your car won't crank. Next, for each barrier you noted, come up with a way you might be able to overcome that barrier. What could you do instead or differently in support of your intellectual self-care? Based on what you came up with, complete the following sentence in your notebook: *Even if or when (insert barrier), I will still (insert clear intention to act in support of intellectual self-care) because (insert why it is important to you to nurture your intellectual self-care).*

Chapter Highlights

- To help your brain function to the best of its ability for as long as possible, you need to exercise it the same way you would exercise your body.
- Learning more about topics you already enjoy can be a great place to start when you want to stimulate your brain.
- Remembering back to when you were a child is one way to help you rediscover topics that excite you.
- Beginner's mind helps you release judgments, expectations, and predictions about how something will go so that you can focus on what is new about the experience.
- A growth mind-set can support intellectual self-care by helping you be open to learning from failure and challenging yourself mentally.

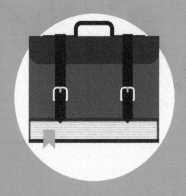

CHAPTER 5

Work & Play
Vocational Self-Care

START HERE IF

Start with vocational self-care if you want to:

→ Find more meaning in your career

→ Use your gifts and talents

→ Establish a connection to your community through volunteer work

→ Improve your level of satisfaction at work

→ Find balance between your work and personal life

Your Vocational Needs

While there are countless ways to earn a living, you will find yourself drawn to some types of work more than others. A vocation is "a strong feeling of suitability for a particular career or occupation." You can think of your vocation as your calling or your life's work. It's work that excites and energizes you. Your vocation is the job you would do for free if you could because it gives you fulfillment—a sense of purpose and meaning.

A vocation is different from a job, because the primary benefit of a job is the paycheck. The benefits of a *vocation* go beyond the things that money can buy to include joy, fulfillment, satisfaction, and passion. Your vocational needs are the types of work, training, and volunteering that you feel especially attracted to, because these activities connect you to a deeper sense of purpose. When you're using your strengths and talents to do work, or volunteering for something meaningful to you, your vocational needs are being met.

While it would be amazing if we all had jobs that we loved and found fulfilling, that's not most people's reality. Work dissatisfaction is at an all-time high in the United States. A recent Gallup survey found that 51 percent of full-time employees in the United States are not engaged at work—they don't believe their work is important and they don't feel personally connected to it; therefore, when they go to work they're "just there," giving minimal effort. This same survey found that 16 percent of employees have a strong dislike for their jobs that leads them to engage in behaviors that ultimately lower morale and overall productivity. The results of this study make clear that work is an area of life where a lot of people feel dissatisfaction.

On top of feeling unhappy at work, people often feel trapped. They feel they don't have enough latitude to make changes because of real-life financial pressures. Even though they're unhappy at work, people feel stuck because they need their paychecks to survive. Another work-related challenge many people face is underemployment. They're in jobs well below what their skill level should earn them, or they can only find part-time work despite wanting a full-time position. Another segment of the population struggles with unemployment. Despite having valuable knowledge, talents, or skills, depending on where they live and outside factors like the strength of the national economy, many people struggle to secure consistent work at all.

Despite all these challenges to having a satisfying work life, there is hope. There are actions you can take—both at work and outside of it—to help you feel as though your vocational self-care needs are being met.

How Do You Want to Contribute to the World?

From eradicating poverty to spreading knowledge to alleviating human suffering, there are various unmet (or under-met) needs in our society that offer opportunities to volunteer or otherwise contribute.

This next activity leads you through a series of questions to answer in your notebook. These will help you better understand what societal needs resonate most with you and the kind of contributions you might like to make. Keep in mind that no contribution is too small. The goal is to make an impact that helps you feel like you're leaving the world a better place than you found it.

1. Think back to your childhood and teen years. Consider the people you knew, the places you played, studied, and gathered.
   - What challenges did members of your family face? What concerns did they discuss?
   - What needs were unmet in your community? In what ways was your environment lacking?
   - What did you or the people around you wish they had more of? Less of?
   - What problems did you become aware of?
   - What news stories did you discuss with your parents or peers?
   - What types of volunteer activities did you participate in?
   - What social problems did you learn about in school that made you want to "do something"?

2. Now think of yourself today. Answer the following questions based on your interests and observations as an adult.
   - What challenges do you and your family face? What keeps you or those you love from realizing your full potential?
   - What needs are unmet in your community? In what ways is your environment lacking?
   - What do you or the people around you long to have more of? Less of?
   - What problems do you hear constantly discussed on social media or in the news?
   - What news stories do you discuss with your family and friends?
   - What types of volunteer activities do you participate in?
   - What problems do you wish you had the time and resources to "do something" about?
   - What issues keep you up at night?

3. Review your answers. Rate how much each issue, need, challenge, or activity appeals to you on a scale of 1 to 10, where 1 is not at all appealing and 10 is extremely appealing. This will help boil down your unique vocational interests.

Now that you've identified the societal needs that resonate with you and you have an idea of how you could make an impact in that area, you might be thinking, "Great, she's asking me to add something else to my already too-full schedule. I don't have time to do more!" You're right; you may not have the time now. What I'm asking is that, rather than add more meaningless tasks to your pile of responsibilities, you start choosing to spend your time engaged in activities that mean something to you. When we spend our time volunteering or doing other activities that benefit others, we feel healthier and happier.

Engage

We've all heard some version of the saying, "Nothing worth having comes easy." This rings true in all areas of our lives, and especially in the vocational realm. Exercising self-care in this area can be extra challenging, particularly if you're one of the many people who feels dissatisfied at work.

If we want to experience more pleasure, joy, meaning, and purpose in the work that we do, it will take effort—whether it's our dream job or not. To improve our lives at work, we need to be actively engaged with our jobs and find ways to make work matter to us. This might include cultivating a positive mind-set about our work environment and the challenges it presents—seeing difficulties and potential roadblocks as opportunities for personal growth. It could also involve making a concerted effort to get better quality sleep so that we can think more clearly at work or build healthier relationships with coworkers so that we feel supported and valued in the workplace.

Where to Start: Weigh the Pros and the Cons

Just like there are no perfect jobs, it's likely the case that no job is 100 percent awful. There is bound to be at least one aspect of your work that you like or appreciate. Maybe you enjoy the short commute you're lucky enough to have. Perhaps you like the support and encouragement you get from your coworkers. Or maybe you enjoy having an interesting job that provides a range of tasks and allows you to put your skills to good use.

Grab your notebook and write down the pros and cons of your current employment situation. Be as specific as possible when describing both and try to spend the same amount of time considering both sides. Here's an example:

Pros: What I Like/Appreciate About My Current Employment Situation	Cons: What I Dislike About My Current Employment Situation
My boss understands the importance of family and has allowed me to leave work early for family emergencies.	Every day is the same—I get bored because I do the same tasks every day, and I am not challenged.

Chances are you've discovered that there are many good aspects of your job, even if they aren't monumental. Focus on the pros and look at the cons as challenges you might be able to find a solution to. The next exercise can help you with that.

Try Something New: Shift Your Focus

It can be easy to complain about work when we're not happy. And don't get me wrong, your feelings and experience are completely valid. I'm sure you have good reasons for feeling the way you feel. I'd be the last to tell you that you shouldn't feel the way you're feeling or that you should keep those feelings bottled up. But it's also the case that constantly broadcasting your dislike or grievance with your job is not likely to make you feel better about your situation. You're already unhappy; why make yourself miserable by constantly focusing your attention on all the things you don't like about your job?

As a first step to taking a more balanced perspective, try this: Next time you find yourself mentally revisiting, for example, the argument you had with your coworker last week, stop and challenge yourself to shift perspectives. Instead, focus on the positive relationship you have with the coworker you *are* friendly with. What you focus on grows in magnitude. If you want to feel more of the emotions that argument brought up, then keep thinking about it. But, if you want to feel differently, shift your focus. Remember, self-care is about engaging in actions that leave you feeling healthy and energized. To help you see what this might look like, go back to your list of pros and cons. Using those as your starting point, I have two challenges for you:

1. **Be thankful for the pros.** During your commute home from work, reflect on your day and silently say one thing you are grateful for that happened at work that day, even if it's just that you are happy to have a job. Do this consistently every day.

2. **Think creatively about ways you can address the cons.** For example, if one of your cons is that you do not feel like you are doing work that makes a difference or gives you a sense of accomplishment, what are some other ways you can get that need met outside of work? Perhaps you could consider volunteering or develop a side hustle—earn money by doing something you are passionate about outside of your typical day job.

Making the Time: Do This, Not That

Like anything worth having in life, enhancing your vocational life requires time and attention. If what's been missing in your life is engaging in work or volunteer activities that give you a sense of accomplishment, meaning, or purpose, then it might be time to build in some activities that fulfill this need for you. While it would be great to have your work meet this need, it just might not be realistic for you right now.

A few years back, David Zinczenko and Matt Goulding wrote *Eat This, Not That!* to help guide Americans looking to make healthier food selections by swapping out high-fat and sugary foods for healthier choices that meet the same need—a kind of one-to-one trade-off system. I suggest a similar strategy for helping you make time for vocational self-care. For instance, the next time you plan to sit down to watch TV or a movie, why not watch a YouTube video demonstrating a skill or technique you've been wanting to master instead? Or the next time you grab your phone and your finger is itching to tap a social media app, why not go to your Internet browser and search for volunteer opportunities in your community?

Expand

It is healthy to have a mixture of work and play in your life. Many of us think of play or hobbies as things we do purely for the fun of it or to avoid boredom, but recreation and hobbies have more than fun to offer. They contribute to vocational self-care by fulfilling us, giving us a sense of purpose even if it's just a matter of completing a creative project or participating in a game. They also help make us smarter, more patient, and better problem solvers. They expand our creativity and self-confidence, and enhance our ability to be in the present moment. They provide us with a sense of happiness, accomplishment, and fulfillment in much the same way as working in a vocation we find meaningful.

Use Hobbies and Play to Improve Your Quality of Life

Many of us look to friends, family, spouses, and work to find happiness and a sense of accomplishment. Sometimes we can get these needs met through these sources, but other times the people in our lives and the work we do fall short of giving us all the passion and fulfillment we long for.

Participating in hobbies and engaging in playful activities are great ways to take responsibility for your own happiness, instead of leaving it in the hands of another person, place, or event. On a scale from 1 to 10, with 1 being the least and 10 being the most, how would you rate your level of happiness and fulfillment? If you chose a rating less than 10, consider how you might take responsibility for improving that number by taking up a hobby or other activity that brings you a sense of joy and accomplishment. Grab your notebook and answer these questions:

- What makes you happy?
- When was the last time you felt capable and talented?
- How might you be able to create the joy and fulfillment you need for yourself?

Expand your horizons—and your happiness level—by identifying something that will bring you a sense of accomplishment, and then take one step toward working that hobby or activity into your life.

Restore

Although many of us have bought into the notion that we should be hustling, hurried, and productive every waking minute, working all the time actually isn't good for us—or for our long-term productivity. Not only is constant work hard on us psychologically, we are actually less effective workers when we don't take breaks—both throughout the day, on weekends, and during vacation time. Also, when we spend more hours working we are prone to prioritize things that matter less—such as our status in the workplace or pulling together a flawless presentation—above the things that matter most, like family and friends, and become addicted to productivity in the process.

Schedule Breaks Throughout Your Day

One of the easiest ways to schedule breaks throughout the day is to build them around your eating schedule. In America, we have a shared cultural expectation of having three meals per day: breakfast, lunch, and dinner. In much the same way, you can create a routine for yourself where you take time to intentionally pause in the morning, at noon, and in the evening. Taking breaks during the workday enhances your vocational self-care because it rejuvenates and reenergizes you.

To schedule regular breaks, start by pegging them to mealtimes—the natural breaks in many people's daily schedules. Start with a small chunk of time—say five minutes—and devote those minutes to something that will restore and rejuvenate you. Examples are a walk around the block, a short breathing exercise, or a guided meditation from a smartphone app.

Remember, this is your break time. Set up a schedule that works best for you. If you only have 30-minute breaks and need 20 minutes to eat, that's fine. Come up with a plan for how you will use the remaining 10 minutes to give yourself extra nourishment, whether that's reading a few pages from a book, listening to music, or meditating.

Protect Your Weekends

With our smartphones making us so accessible by phone, text, or e-mail, we've grown accustomed to working at least a little bit on the weekends, checking e-mail, or responding to texts. Working on the weekends can make us feel like we're being productive and getting ahead, because there always seems to be more work than there is time to do it. The truth is, there will always be more work to do and you cannot do it all.

Think about it: The last time you pulled an all-nighter or skipped your child's sporting event to catch up on work, did you really check everything off your to-do list? It's likely that even if you did everything you wanted to do that day, there were still other work-related tasks you could have done but chose to save for another day.

Actually, taking a break from your work on the weekend allows you time to mentally recharge, and space to come up with fresh ideas and new ways of tackling work-related challenges. Even if you only pick one weekend day to preserve, you will still benefit. Here are some tips for protecting your weekends:

- Avoid sharing your personal cell phone number with your boss.
- Avoid checking work-related e-mail.
- Let your coworkers know that you don't generally work on weekends.
- Turn off your smartphone alerts.
- Preplan weekend activities with family and friends.
- Preplan "me time" weekend activities.
- Preplan a weekend getaway or "staycation" with your spouse or friend.

Reward Yourself

As a reward for prioritizing your vocational self-care, invest in yourself by buying or doing something that makes you feel cared for. Some people find spending money on themselves challenging because it may seem unwise or selfish when there's a pile of financial responsibilities. But self-care is *not* selfish; it's about giving to yourself so that you have reserves of energy available to make a difference in the lives of others. Author Eleanor Brownn summed it up best with this quote: "Rest and self-care are so important. When you take time to replenish your spirit, it allows you to serve others from the overflow. You cannot serve from an empty vessel." Taking care of yourself is the key to being the best version of you.

Grow

No matter where you are in your career, it's always a good idea to keep growing, learning, and developing new skills. Developing new skills can help increase your earning potential at your current job, position you to move from part-time to full-time employment, or lay the foundation for new employment that's closer to what you feel is your real calling. When you are in an employment situation that is less than ideal, focusing on developing skills you can take with you to another job can help make your current situation feel more comfortable.

Areas for Growth

A great place to start when challenging yourself to grow in your work life is to consider what skills you'd like to develop or strengthen. Take a look back at "How Do You Want to Contribute to the World?" (see page 79). Based on the items you ranked highest in your notebook, make a list of all the skills and resources you might need to pursue those activities. Next, note whether you already have those skills or resources or need to obtain them. Finally, make a plan for how you could realistically acquire the skills or resources that are new to you (remember SMART goals; see page 69). How could you use your free moments throughout the day, in the evenings, and on weekends to gain the skills or resources you need to make the impact you want to have on the world?

I'll give you an example of how I set these kinds of goals in my own life. One of my vocational values is to use my mental health knowledge and personal experiences to inspire others to overcome life's challenges and realize their full potential. I'd like to make this impact through speaking engagements at women's empowerment conferences and retreats. Some of the skills and resources I need to do this include the ability to craft engaging messages, public speaking skills, marketing skills to publicize myself as a speaker, video recordings of myself speaking, and a list of fees for my speaking services. While I have two of the skills listed, I need to work on crafting engaging messages, video recordings of myself speaking, and a list of fees. To learn how to do these things, I might hire a coach to help me craft fresh messages, spend some time on the Internet researching videographers in my area, and use Microsoft Office to develop a list of fees.

Look at one of your most exciting vocational goals. What strengths will you bring to this endeavor and what skills or resources do you need to obtain? What are some steps you can take to obtain them?

Get the Experience You Need

No matter how much formal education and training you have received, sometimes skills need to be developed through direct experience. There are several ways you might go about acquiring the experience you need to have the impact you want to have in the world. Here are a few ideas for gaining valuable vocational experiences:

- If you want to experience serving a specific population, volunteer at a school, library, or nonprofit organization.

- If you need "on the job" experience, participate in an internship program or ask to shadow someone who has the type of career you want.
- If you want leadership experience, volunteer for a leadership position in your place of worship, a community organization, or at your child's school.
- If you want teaching or public speaking experience, host a free webinar, workshop, or speaking engagement at your local library.

The keys to setting yourself up for success in gaining the experience you need include:

- Being clear and specific about the type of experience you are seeking.
- Asking directly if the organization, person, or event can provide you with the specific experience you are seeking.
- Speaking up if you are not getting the experience that was advertised.
- Being flexible and thinking about ways to make the experience mutually beneficial for you and the organization you are working with.

Bloom Where You're Planted

Regardless of the type or scale of the impact you want to have in the world, unless you are incredibly fortunate, you will encounter times when you're required to do work that's out of sync with your true passion. Or if you are already doing passion work, there are likely some tasks involved that you don't find pleasing. Whenever you find yourself in either of these situations, your mind-set is key. The mind-set you approach your work with can make all the difference in whether your days are filled with drudgery or with optimism. You may not be where you want to be in your work life right now, but you can choose to bloom where you're planted and believe in yourself.

Blooming where you're planted is another way of capturing the sentiment *"Make lemons out of lemonade."* It's about making the most out of a less-than-ideal situation. Here are three steps to blooming where you are planted:

1. **Use your current situation to make you a better person.** Your current situation can provide lots of learning opportunities, if you stay open to them. Instead of counting down the minutes, hours, days, and weeks until you land that dream job, choose to make the most of where you are now. Maybe you can learn how to be more patient when you come in contact with difficult people. Maybe you can learn better time management or organizational skills. Or perhaps you can develop the skill of gratitude—being thankful for what you have, instead of focusing on what you don't like. When you use your current situation to better yourself, you increase the chances that you can show up in the future well equipped to leave your mark on the world.

2. **Leave your workplace better than you found it.** Don't let your current circumstances bring you down. Look for ways to leave a positive impact. Something as simple as a smile or offer of support can leave a lasting impression. What can you do to spread harmony, peace, and kindness to the people you come in contact with daily at work? Instead of admiring someone from afar, give them a compliment. Can you use your voice to speak up for someone who is unable to speak up for themselves? Can you give your undivided attention to the next person you interact with? How about offering to help someone in need without being asked? Don't underestimate your power. Simple gestures can have a great impact.

3. **Never stop dreaming.** Just because your current situation isn't ideal doesn't mean it will always be that way. Have faith that better days are ahead. Start planning and taking small actions that move you closer to your ideal work situation. Start small, do what you can with what you have, and trust that your small acts of faith will be rewarded.

Believe in Yourself and Make an Impact

When we dream big and want to have an impact on the world, it can seem as though we are too small or insignificant to make a true impact. Consider the following: "If you think you're too small to make a difference, you haven't spent a night with a mosquito." I love this proverb because it reminds me that, even as an army of one, I am a capable and powerful force to be reckoned with. Sometimes we just need a little reminder of how capable, resilient, and awesome we are. The next time you need a little inspiration to believe in yourself, listen to a song or read a poem or quote that makes you feel empowered.

A perfect example of an "army of one" is Mother Teresa. She said, "Do small things with great love." The way Mother Teresa lived her life is a testament to the power of one. Take a look back at "How Do You Want to Contribute to the World?" (see page 79). Identify the activity you ranked the highest. What one small action can you commit to taking in the next week that moves you closer to having the impact you want to have in your family, community, or the world? Commit to taking your small action with great love—for yourself and others.

Chapter Highlights

- Your vocational needs are being met when you are using your strengths and talents to do work that you feel has meaning and purpose, whether or not you are paid for it.
- If you want to experience more pleasure, joy, meaning, and purpose in the work you do, you may need to change your focus from the cons to the pros.
- Although many of us have bought into the notion that we should be hustling, hurried, and productive every waking minute, working all the time isn't good for you.
- No matter where you are in your career, it is never a bad idea to continue growing, learning, and developing new skills.
- The mind-set with which you approach your work can make all the difference in whether your days are filled with complete misery or hopeful expectation.

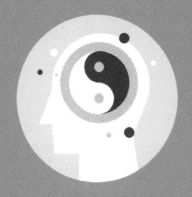

CHAPTER **6**

Your Higher Self
Spiritual Self-Care

START HERE IF

Start with spiritual self-care if you want to:

→ Learn what spirituality means to you

→ Deepen your faith and calm your mind

→ Quiet the external voices long enough to hear your own voice and intuition

→ Find perspective beyond the hustle and bustle of daily life

→ Enrich your connection with a higher power

→ Discover or reconnect to what matters most to you

→ Fulfill your craving for spiritual nourishment

→ Connect with a community that shares your spiritual practices

Your Spiritual Needs

Beneath everything you see when you look in the mirror—your hair, your clothes, your physical appearance—there is something more. Some people call it your soul; others call it spirit. The particular words don't matter as much as understanding that your spirit, as I'm going to call it, represents the essence of who you are.

When all the labels, roles, titles, and possessions have been stripped away, your spirit is what remains. It's been there all along; from the moment you exited the womb, the essence of *you* was there. And as you have journeyed through life—facing joys, disappointments, and changes—the essence of who you are has remained the same. The energy you bring into a room, your likes and dislikes, your passion, the various emotions you experience, your intellect and creativity, all combine to characterize your nonmaterial, fundamental self.

Spiritual self-care revolves around engaging in activities that turn our attention inward and reconnect us with ourselves. Spiritual self-care helps us cultivate a deeper sense of clarity about what matters most to us and what we believe in. We take care of our spiritual needs by taking time away from the daily grind to get quiet and tune in to our own inner wisdom. It involves connecting to something that is larger than ourselves, like worshipping in a faith community, spending time in nature, seeking guidance through prayer or meditation, practicing yoga, journaling, or spending time in personal reflection. Tending to our spiritual self-care is less about believing in a higher power, and more about recognizing that we exist and have needs beyond the physical and material realm.

Have you ever felt a hunger for more fulfillment in life that just didn't seem to be satisfied by material things? That hunger is probably a sign of an unmet spiritual need. Psychologist Abraham Maslow famously said that all humans have five different types of needs:

1. Physiological (food, water, sleep, and shelter)

2. Safety

3. Love and belonging

4. Esteem

5. Self-actualization (becoming the best version of one's self)

He suggested that the needs have a ranked order, where the ones at the bottom (physiological, safety, and love/belonging) are the most fundamental and need to be fulfilled before we can focus our energy on the ones at the top (esteem and self-actualization).

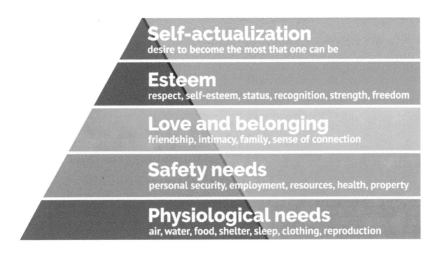

Our spiritual needs can be likened to the highest-level need of personal development. They are those longings that remain once the more basic physical and emotional needs have been satisfied. Spiritual needs propel us to put our talents to good use for the betterment of the people and the world around us. Connecting with our spiritual needs brings us closer to the "higher calling" so many of us are seeking.

How Do You Want to Be Remembered?

Our time on Earth is short. We don't like to talk about it much in our society, but we're confronted with the reality of our mortality every time we hear about fatalities on the news, look in the mirror and notice a gray hair, or watch a loved one battle a serious illness.

Rather than avoid the inevitable, what would it be like if we acknowledged our fragility? I was reminded of this recently when I received the devastating news that one of my students—just 21 years old and full of promise—had died in a car accident. After the initial shock wore off, I began to ponder my student's life and legacy. I wondered, "When she's remembered by family and friends, what will they say about her? What did her life represent? What did she stand for?" Then the reality hit that I, too, will eventually face my final days. Just as my student is now remembered in death, I will one day only be a memory.

The question that kept coming up for me was, "What do I want people to say about me when I'm gone?" It wasn't an easy question to sit with, because I realized that, despite my best intentions, I don't always behave in ways I want to be remembered for. I'd like to be remembered as someone who made an impact, but sometimes I let the fear of what others will say, or fear of failure, stop me from working to leave my mark on the world. I suspect most people can relate to this. Maybe there are things you want to stand for in life, but sometimes you fall short of the expectations you have for yourself. The good news is, we get an endless supply of do-overs in life. We get a fresh start each minute. A favorite poem of mine touches on this theme. It's by an unknown author, but was frequently cited by Dr. Benjamin E. Mays—it's titled "I Have Only Just a Minute":

> *I have only just a minute,*
> *Only sixty seconds in it*
> *Forced upon me, can't refuse it.*
> *Didn't seek it, didn't choose it.*
> *But it's up to me*
> *to use it.*
> *I must suffer if I lose it.*
> *Give account if I abuse it.*
> *Just a tiny little minute,*
> *but eternity is in it.*

I love this poem because it reminds me that it's never too late to be who I want to be, to start doing the kinds of things I want to be remembered for. My invitation to you is to consider how you want to be remembered. For generations to come, what do you want people to say you stood for? In your notebook, complete the following sentence: *I stand for (insert value), (insert value), and (insert value)*.

If you need some assistance, here is a list of spiritual values for inspiration, but don't be limited by it:

Spiritual Values

Abundance	Gentleness	Love
Acceptance	Goodness	Loyalty
Authenticity	Gratitude	Passion
Balance	Honesty	Peace
Compassion	Humility	Righteousness
Consistency	Humor	Sacrifice
Creativity	Inspiration	Self-Control
Discernment	Integrity	Strength
Faith	Joy	Trust
Faithfulness	Justice	Understanding
Forbearance	Kindness	Vitality
Forgiveness	Liberation	Wisdom
Generosity		

Engage

Spiritual self-care is important because it can help us make sense of the hurt and pain we experience in our lives. We all know pain. It's an inevitable part of the human experience. Whether our pain originates from loss, rejection, betrayal, loneliness, disappointment, failure, or a physical injury, it can turn our lives upside down, leaving complex layers of emotional scars that interfere with our ability to experience joy and pleasure.

Our spiritual beliefs give us a lens through which to view our pain. Spiritual beliefs help us make sense of the hard places we land in life, and they can offer us hope when the pain is great and life seems unfair. Spiritual self-care helps us develop a deeper relationship with ourselves; it reacquaints us with the beliefs and practices that bring us peace and perspective when the going gets rough.

Where to Start: Sit Still and Be Quiet

Getting to know yourself on a deeper, more spiritual level requires you to be still long enough to hear your own voice. It can be challenging to hear your own inner voice when you are receiving outside perspectives from family, friends, coworkers, television, and magazines. Listening to your own inner voice helps you reconnect with the truth of who you are and what really matters most to you. Your inner voice can be a subtle guide that helps you make challenging decisions.

To help get you familiar with your inner wisdom, intentionally set aside five minutes each day to just be quiet. Don't distract yourself with anything. Just simply sit, either indoors or in nature, in stillness and quiet. Afterward, spend a few minutes journaling in your notebook about what showed up for you during those moments of stillness.

Try Something New: Be of Service

Serving others supports our spiritual self-care by helping us feel connected to other people and causes that are larger than us, distracting us from our own problems and buffering against the stress and anxiety we are confronted with on a daily basis. There are many ways to be of service. It can be as simple as buying a coffee for the person behind you in the Starbucks line, volunteering, or donating money to a charity of your choosing. Being of service is all about meeting the needs of someone else, seeking justice for marginalized populations, or speaking on behalf of someone who cannot freely speak for themselves.

Grab your notebook and answer the following questions:

- What needs have you seen in your community lately?
- What cause or issue are you passionate about?
- How might you use your time, talent, or resources to be of service in that area?

Once you've spent some time exploring your answers to these questions, consider one action you can take to nurture yourself in the domain of spiritual self-care.

Making the Time: Start Small

Opening time in your schedule for spiritual self-care doesn't need to start with memorizing the Bible, going on a spiritual retreat, or attending a worship service every week. It also doesn't require that you meditate or pray first thing in the morning every day. Sure, these might be goals you can work toward, but don't be afraid to start small with spiritual self-care.

You'd be surprised at what taking five minutes out of your day for spiritual self-care can do for your spirit. Simply taking a few minutes to meditate, say a prayer, read an uplifting blog, or spend time in nature can give you the spiritual boost you need to remain calm and connected to your inner voice. It really doesn't take a huge chunk of your time to make a big difference. Consider your upcoming week and think of ways to feed your spirit for just five minutes. When you're ready, you can add more time to your spiritual self-care routine if you'd like to.

Center

One step you can take toward greater clarity and inner peace is learning how to center yourself. Centering yourself involves training yourself to maintain focus on what matters most in the midst of stressful situations. When we are stressed, our minds shower us with a downpour of negative thoughts, we are flooded with overwhelming emotions, and our bodies become containers of tension, ready to blow at any given moment.

Centering helps you stay calm and grounded when you are feeling overwhelmed or afraid. Much like lowering the temperature of a pot of water at full flame before it boils over, we need strategies to help calm ourselves when we're feeling overwhelmed and anxious.

Centering helps us regain perspective in the midst of chaos, and transform anxiety into calm, positive energy.

Take a Breath

Our breath is a built-in relaxation system that can help us find calm in the midst of any situation. We just have to be willing to pause and tune in to it. Make a mental note that the next time you are feeling anxious, stressed, or uncertain, you will turn to your breath to regain your calm.

As soon as you notice that you are feeling tense and over-whelmed, focus on the rise and fall of your belly. Just take a moment to feel your belly breathing. As you inhale, notice the sensations of your stomach stretching each time you breathe in and shrinking each time you breathe out. When anxious thoughts arise, see if it's possible to let them fade into the background of your awareness and keep focusing on the breath. After five deep belly breaths, check in with yourself. How do you feel?

Meet Your Needs

It's hard to tap into your center when other, more basic needs haven't been met. Many times, we are prone to feeling overwhelmed, stuck, or anxious because we have a need we haven't taken care of. If you haven't taken care of your own inner needs, you will be more prone to anxiety, irritability, and stress, and it's hard to do anything effectively when you're not feeling okay.

In my own life, I'm prone to feeling overwhelmed when I'm hungry. I can't seem to focus on anything, and I'm much less tolerant of annoyances. Left unchecked, my hunger quickly affects my mood, leaving me vulnerable to irritability and full-blown anger. I get down-right "hangry"! As soon as I eat, "hangry Robyn" disappears, my focus is restored, and my capacity for patience and kindness quickly returns.

The next time you're feeling overwhelmed by emotions, check in with yourself and see if there are any unmet needs that require your attention. Perhaps you are hungry, tired, burned out, or maybe you have a headache. Get yourself a glass of water (dehydration is a common cause of headaches) and see what needs, physical or otherwise, might be unmet in that moment. Taking care of this need can help redirect your energy and focus to the present moment, allowing you to tap into your own inner wisdom and use it to guide your actions.

Transcend

Our spiritual needs are those that transcend the material—for example, the need to feel valued, connected, and capable. By focusing on our nonmaterial needs, we learn to encounter day-to-day worries, disappointments, and anxieties without becoming consumed by them. This ability to hold our experience lightly keeps us functioning better and is a big part of our ability to recover quickly from difficulties rather than being irreparably broken by them.

One thing that can help keep you from getting too caught up in the troubles of daily life is having a mind-set that recognizes that, because you exist beyond the physical, you are greater than any one experience you will ever have. Whether the experience is a betrayal, loss, or deep disappointment, it is always smaller than you are—and the feelings triggered by even a devastating event are always temporary. Just like a fireplace is sturdy enough to withstand the scorching temperatures of a blazing fire, you are capable of withstanding the deepest of pain and disappointments.

We see examples of the resilience of the human spirit all around us. It's in the mother who had a miscarriage yet was brave enough to try for a child again. The well-adjusted adult who, despite years of childhood abuse and neglect, overcame the odds to live a successful life. We see extreme resilience in our military personnel who face horrific casualties during their term of service yet are able to reintegrate back into civilian life. A part of what makes these individuals resilient is their willingness to face, and then rise above, these difficult experiences.

Don't Believe Everything You Think

Part of the ability to transcend present circumstances rests in your willingness to change your relationship with your thoughts and feelings. A burden is lifted when you recognize that your feelings are only temporary, and your thoughts do not always reflect the reality of your situation. For example, how many times have you heard someone recounting a story of when they had to do something stressful like fly on a plane despite a severe fear of heights or give a public speech and they said, "I literally thought I was going to die!" Obviously, they didn't actually die because they lived to tell the story. And I would imagine that as they are telling the story, they don't feel like they are going to die. But that doesn't mean they didn't feel extreme emotions during that anxiety-provoking situation.

Sometimes thoughts and emotions can appear more dangerous and threatening than reality. Because of this, it's not always wise to allow our thoughts and emotions to dictate our actions. Our emotions will urge us to get rid of emotional pain by any means necessary, but "by any means necessary" is not always what is best for us. If we are not careful, we can create a life where we are imprisoned by our thoughts and feelings—living for comfort, avoiding pain and anxiety, but never really experiencing anything deeply meaningful or pleasurable.

When I work with a client who experiences sudden panic attacks that don't appear to have a specific trigger, I often hear the real terror in their voice as they describe their experience during an attack. They recount the intense body sensations of muscle tension, sweaty palms, upset stomach, chest tightness, shallow breathing, and a fast heartbeat. The rapid heartbeat that most people experience during a panic attack is often interpreted by their brain as a heart attack. Their thoughts tell them that they are having a heart attack, and this thought compels them to visit the emergency room convinced that what their mind told them was true: They are having a heart attack.

My clients who have had this experience reported that they were caught completely off guard when, after being examined by an ER physician, they learn that their thoughts deceived them. Even though their minds told them they were having a life-threatening heart attack, in reality their lives were not in danger. Their symptoms were not indicative of a heart attack. It was just very real and intense anxiety. Like those who experience extreme panic attacks, we are all susceptible to being deceived by our thoughts. Our thoughts have the power to determine our actions. If we are not careful, our thoughts can lead us into deep despair, convincing us that there is no hope.

To help us manage stress and make better decisions when we are feeling overwhelmed, we must learn how to take control of our thoughts and feelings, rather than allowing them to boss us around, controlling whether or not we experience joy and happiness. We do this by learning to observe them. When we observe our thoughts and feelings, we watch them come and go. We allow them to exist within us without attaching to them. Just like typing on a computer, we can watch as various alerts pop up on the screen without getting too attached to each notification. We can watch our thoughts and feelings arise and fall without doing anything about them.

By observing your thoughts, you can detach from what they are telling you long enough to consider whether what they are telling you is real and true. Observing your thoughts and feelings allows you to use your inner wisdom to determine whether your thoughts and feelings are leading you on a path that aligns with your deeper values and goals. The skill of observing can protect you from mindlessly making choices that offer immediate relief or gratification but do not ultimately move you closer to becoming the type of person you want to be. To help you develop this ability, download the Insight Timer app and practice the "You Are Not Your Thoughts Meditation" by StressFit or "Mindfulness of Thoughts and Emotions Practice" by Sara Rabinovitch, Ph.D. The easiest way to locate these meditations is to search the app for the author's name (StressFit or Sara Rabino-vitch), and then look for all guided meditations by that author.

Another way you can learn to observe your thoughts is to be intentional about how you speak *about* your thoughts. For example, when you have the thought, "I am a failure," instead of accepting the label of being a failure, say, "I am having the thought that I am a fail-ure." Just this simple change in language can help you detach from the thought and recognize it for what it is: a thought, rather than an indisputable truth.

> ## Reward Yourself
>
> Reward yourself for prioritizing your spiritual self-care by buying a new journal or fancy ink pen that you can use to express your deepest desires, thoughts, and feelings. Start with these journaling prompts: "What is the best gift I can give myself today?" and "In this moment, what words does my spiritual self need to hear?"

Grow

One of the reasons spiritual self-care can be so challenging is that it's not as tangible as other domains like physical self-care. No matter who you are, exercise is good for you, but there is no one-size-fits-all strategy for fulfilling our spiritual longings. Our spiritual needs are unique to us, and it can take a while for us to get clear about what gives our life meaning and purpose.

Spiritual growth is not always direct. Sometimes spiritual beliefs change and evolve as we grow, and our spiritual needs change along with our beliefs. Spiritual growth is a journey without a final destination. One of the ways to make the journey easier is to connect with people who have similar spiritual values and aspirations. It can be beneficial to practice spiritual self-care in community settings. A second way to make the journey of spiritual self-care easier is by protecting our peace of mind. We can do this by avoiding toxicity (for example, unhealthy relationships or overconsumption of upsetting stories in the media) and controlling where we focus our attention and who we spend time with.

Find Your Tribe

Once you have done some of the inner work required to gain clarity about your personal spiritual beliefs, find a group of people who will practice spiritual self-care alongside you and support you as you continue to grow spiritually. You might find your tribe by attending a place of worship or a spiritual community service, exploring nature with fellow nature lovers, attending a weekly meditation group, connecting with others by sharing your spiritual beliefs on a community blog, or reading spiritual texts in a Bible study or book club setting.

Protect Your Peace

We can maintain a peaceful spirit in the midst of anxiety, worry, and uncertainty if we keep our mind focused on thoughts, images, and memories that help us feel calm. Keeping your mind in peace might also require you to temporarily avoid things, people, and content that don't make you feel peaceful. To protect my peace, I find it beneficial to take occasional breaks from social media. While social media platforms provide a great opportunity to connect with others, they also fuel perfectionism and comparison. People rarely post the struggles they have on social media. We'll snap 50 (or more!) selfies just to get that one "Instagram-worthy" picture. When we're going through our own personal struggles, seeing everyone else's perfectly scripted life on social media can intensify our pain by causing us to compare ourselves and convincing us that everyone else has it all together. We end up feeling inadequate and alone in our struggles.

Taking a break from social media is one of many ways you can protect your peace. You can also protect your peace by being intentional about the thoughts you focus on, the shows you watch on television, the type of music you listen to, and the people you surround yourself with. Although you can't protect yourself from life's troubles, you can set yourself up to experience peace in the midst of troubles by being intentional about what you consume. Get out your notebook and take some time to brainstorm actions you can take to protect your peace.

What Will You Do with Your One Life?

Look back at what you wrote in your notebook while completing the "How Do You Want to Be Remembered?" exercise (see page 95). You identified three values you want to be remembered for. Pick one of those values to focus on today.

What one action can you do today that will help you be remembered the way you want to be remembered? Keep in mind that there's no shame in starting small; just start with intentionality and an open heart. Our spiritual beliefs provide a lens through which to filter the hard circumstances of life. They help us have hope and faith when life gets hard. Find an object or picture that reminds you to have faith and put it in a location where you will see it daily.

Chapter Highlights

- Your spirit is the essence of who you are. When all the labels, roles, and titles have been stripped away, your spirit is what remains.
- Spiritual self-care helps you develop a deeper sense of clarity about what matters most to you and what you believe to be true. Taking time away from the daily grind to get quiet and listen for your inner wisdom nourishes your spirit.
- Simply taking five minutes to say a prayer, meditate, read a spiritually uplifting blog, or go outside and be in nature can give you the spiritual boost you need to remain calm and connected to your inner voice. It doesn't take a huge chunk of your time to make a big difference.
- Your spiritual beliefs give you a lens through which to view your pain. Spiritual beliefs help you make sense of the hard places you may land in life, and they can offer hope when pain is unrelenting and life seems unfair.
- Centering yourself helps you stay calm and grounded when you are feeling overwhelmed or afraid.
- Part of the ability to transcend present circumstances rests in your willingness to change your relationship with your thoughts and feelings. Recognize that your feelings are temporary and your thoughts do not always reflect the reality of your situation.
- Spiritual growth is a journey without a final destination.

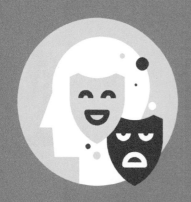

CHAPTER 7

Be Your Own Best Friend
Emotional Self-Care

START HERE IF

Start with emotional self-care if you want to:

→ Strengthen your ability to manage difficult emotions

→ Stop avoiding your feelings

→ Expand your tolerance for emotional pain

→ Be less reactive when you experience intense emotions

→ Respond effectively when your feelings are being dismissed or invalidated by others

→ Learn your emotional triggers

→ Take care of yourself when you are experiencing emotional pain

Your Emotional Needs

Have you ever wondered why we have emotions? What purpose is served by feeling angry, happy, frightened, or confident? Many of my clients have had this same question. For many, emotions are a source of seemingly unrelenting pain. Emotions can make us feel like we're on an unpredictable roller coaster that vacillates between thrilling heights and heart-sinking lows that keep us bracing on the edge of our seat, just waiting for the next drop. What's the point of it all?

Well, emotions actually help us accomplish quite a bit. The number one reason we have emotions is because they help us survive. Imagine if you were able to stare a roaring lion in the face without feeling one ounce of fear. Without fear, you would not be motivated to engage in self-protective behaviors like running away. Emotions help ensure our survival by motivating us to engage in behaviors that keep us safe. A second reason we have emotions is that they help us take inspired action and make decisions. The anxiety you feel when you are about to give a presentation at work or take a test at school can motivate you to prepare and increase your chances for success. Third, emotions allow us to communicate effectively with others. Because of emotions, we can read our children's nonverbal expressions of sadness and respond supportively. Similarly, emotions allow us to communicate to others how we feel in the midst of a heated debate or a moment of extreme passion. Our ability to communicate how we feel—and read the emotions of others—helps us understand each other and respond appropriately.

I like the way author Lysa TerKeurst describes the purpose of emotional pain. In her book *It's Not Supposed to Be This Way*, she writes, "The feeling of the pain is like a warning light on the dashboard of our car. The light comes on to indicate something is wrong. We can assume it's a little glitch in the operating panel. We can even go to the mechanic and ask him to turn off that annoying little light. But if he's a good mechanic, he would tell you it's foolish not to pay attention to it. Because if you don't attend to it, you will soon experience a breakdown. The warning light isn't trying to annoy you. It's trying to protect you." Just like painful emotions are a signal telling us that something needs attention, pleasant emotions can also signal us to pay attention and embrace the simple pleasures in life.

Simply stated, our emotions help us notice things that need our attention. Emotional self-care involves acknowledging and embracing all of our emotions—both pleasant and unpleasant feelings—and giving ourselves what we need when we are experiencing emotional pain. It requires self-awareness and time for reflection. Emotional self-care also requires a willingness to hold emotions lightly—to not get too attached to a particular emotional state (whether good or bad) and allow emotions to come and go.

Emotional self-care can help us manage daily stress and mental health challenges (anxiety or depression, for example). Emotional self-care can also help us heal from traumatic experiences, like physical abuse and neglect, and adverse childhood experiences such as having witnessed domestic violence and crime. We can engage in emotional self-care on our own, in the form of self-help, but remember that it can often benefit us to seek support from a qualified mental health professional.

What Relationship Do You Want to Have with Your Feelings?

There are three types of relationships we can have with our feelings: passive, aggressive, or assertive. Let's take a look at each:

- **Passive.** When we are passive with our feelings, we become enslaved to them, simply going along with whatever they urge us to do. We relinquish any influence we might have on our emotions.
- **Aggressive.** When we are aggressive with our emotions, we insist that they be better or different, and we approach changing our emotions with a "by any means necessary" approach. When we have an aggressive relationship with our emotions, we find it difficult to make space for painful emotions, and we may even harm ourselves physically or emotionally to avoid feeling emotional pain.
- **Assertive.** When we have an assertive relationship with our emotions, we are willing to have uncomfortable emotions. When

we are hurting, we gently embrace the pain, recognizing that it won't always be like this. We are willing to say how we really feel, whether or not it makes other people uncomfortable. When we experience positive emotions, we allow ourselves to savor those moments while not clinging on to them too tightly. When we have an assertive relationship with our emotions, although we cannot control our emotions, we recognize that we do have the power to influence our feelings. We know, ultimately, that we control how we respond when feeling emotional, and we take the initiative to set up our environment in a way that helps us cope effectively.

Consider these descriptions and ask yourself what type of relationship you currently have with your emotions. Then, in your notebook, identify what type of relationship you *want* to have with your emotions. Where do you see opportunities for growth?

Engage

Emotional health means that you have the ability to cope with life's challenges and allow yourself to fully experience a variety of pleasant and unpleasant emotions. Contrary to popular belief, being emotionally healthy doesn't mean that you're happy all the time. An aspect of emotional health is knowing how to manage your emotions in a way that's kind, to you and others. Managing your emotions requires a willingness to be present with the full range of emotions, both pleasant and unpleasant.

Where to Start: Know Your Emotions

When we feel an emotion, it's important to be able to label that emotional experience appropriately. Having words for your experience helps you feel empowered to do something about it—even if that means choosing to simply feel the emotion until it subsides. Not only does having an emotional vocabulary help you understand how you are feeling, it also helps you communicate your emotions to others and read the cues that indicate how other people are feeling.

Developing an emotional vocabulary requires practice. Unfortunately, this skill isn't taught in the traditional U.S. school system, so many of us venture into adulthood lacking the words to express the various emotions we experience. One way to grow your emotional vocabulary is to identify and label emotions you might feel in various situations. Here's a list of emotional trigger scenarios that anyone might encounter in daily life:

Receiving an unexpected compliment.

Getting stuck in traffic on the way to work.

Taking your dog for a walk in beautiful weather.

Reading a book for pleasure.

Receiving news that a loved one has died.

Volunteering for an organization or cause that you are passionate about.

Watching children play at the park.

Running late for an important meeting or appointment.

Eating your favorite food.

Achieving a goal you've been working toward for the past couple of months.

Receiving a warm embrace from a loved one.

Reconnecting with an old friend.

Grab your notebook and write down how you might feel if you experienced each of these situations. If you have trouble coming up with emotions for yourself in each hypothetical situation, imagine that the experience happened to a loved one. Consider how they might feel if they experienced the situation.

For each scenario, challenge yourself to write down at least two emotions: one primary emotion, and one more specific secondary emotion that more accurately captures how you would feel. Some theorists have suggested that the six primary emotions we feel are joyful, fearful, mad, sad, peaceful, and powerful. For example, if someone cut you off in traffic and almost caused an accident, you will likely be angry, but anger has varying levels of intensity. You could be mildly irritated, annoyed, angry, fuming, irate, livid, or furious. Challenging yourself to come up with a more specific description to capture the flavor and intensity of your emotion will help you expand your emotional vocabulary. Feel free to use a thesaurus to help you get more specific.

It's also important to recognize that the same situation can trigger a variety of emotions that seem contradictory. Emotions are like that sometimes. Two emotions that contradict each other can arise at the same time. For example, 2018 was the 10-year anniversary of my father losing his battle with cancer. To celebrate his life and legacy, I planned a gathering for my extended family on my father's side. When I attended this gathering, I felt a combination of emotions. I felt sad that my father wasn't there to celebrate with us, but at the same time, I was happy about the opportunity to reconnect with family members I hadn't seen in years. So, when writing down emotions for each scenario in the exercise, feel free to include contradictory emotions.

Try Something New: Identify Your Triggers

Taking care of yourself emotionally requires self-awareness. It's important to recognize the situations that typically cause you to feel both pleasant and unpleasant emotions. This information can help you anticipate how you might respond to a specific situation, and make a plan to better manage situations or people that you know trigger negative responses.

Over the next week, monitor the connection between your behavior and your mood. At least once each hour, check in with yourself. In your notebook, write down a quick note about your surroundings (the situation) and what you're doing (the behavior), and then write the emotion you are experiencing.

After a week of this, examine your notes and see if you can spot any patterns. This will help you have a better understanding of the types of behaviors and situations that trigger both positive and negative emotions for you. Armed with increased awareness of your triggers, you can enter situations that trigger unwanted emotions with more awareness and care, and also intentionally engage in behaviors that are likely to produce pleasant emotions.

Making the Time: Learn to Say "No"

To prioritize your emotional health, you will need to create time in your daily or weekly schedule to engage in behaviors that support your emotional health. Whether it's journaling your feelings, engaging in self-reflection, or attending a therapy appointment, those activities require time. That means you'll need to prioritize the activities that are most important to you and aligned with your values. Then, you have to be willing to say "no" to the activities, requests, invitations, and offers that you simply do not have time for because they do not fall at the top of your list of priorities. Remember: Even though you would like to do all the things, you simply cannot do them all and do them all well. Something has to give.

It's also important to acknowledge that many of us tend to say yes when we really want to say no. We volunteer for projects, go to meetings, and sign up for tasks that we don't want to do because we want to please others. We don't want to be judged, rejected, or disliked for saying no. The problem is that in the process of putting everyone else's needs first, you're putting yourself on the back burner.

Understand that saying no doesn't make you a bad person. Quite the contrary, it communicates that you are prioritizing your own well-being. Learning to say no is not only a good time-management strategy, but it also nurtures your emotional health by ensuring that you are spending your precious time engaged in the activities that are most important and valuable to you. Your challenge for this week is to look for opportunities to say no. It won't be easy at first, but, as with most things in life, it gets easier with practice. Here are some tips to help you say no with confidence:

- **Say no as soon as you decide to say no.** Keep in mind that the person who asked you will need to find someone else to take your place. Give them adequate time by declining promptly.

- **Be gracious.** Express appreciation for the offer or invitation.
- **Be truthful.** When you make up an excuse for saying no that is not truthful, you're just setting yourself up to feel bad.

What do you do when you really want to say yes but are not sure if you should? This can be hard because although we can do something, it doesn't mean we *should* do it. A simple practice I have adopted is giving myself 24 hours to respond. When I feel the urge to say yes but need to seriously evaluate whether that is the wisest choice for me, giving myself 24 hours helps me to exercise emotional restraint. Here's an example of what I might say in these situations:

Thank you so much for thinking of me for this opportunity. Given my current responsibilities, I want to take some time to consider whether I can give this the time, energy, and effort it deserves. Can I get back to you with an answer in 24 hours?

Then I give myself time to consider the pros and cons of saying yes and the pros and cons of saying no. This helps me make choices that are in line with my values, rather than making an emotion-based decision in the heat of the moment that I might live to regret. I don't always get it right and neither will you, but I am getting better at not letting my initial excitement lead me into making a hasty decision. It just helps to give ourselves some space.

Saying no can be especially challenging for my fellow recovering perfectionists, people pleasers, and conflict avoiders. For us, in addition to evaluating our priorities and the pros and cons, it can be helpful to ask ourselves five questions when we are tempted to say yes:

1. Do I want to do this?

2. Am I trying to gain acceptance or approval from someone else?

3. Am I trying to avoid conflict or keep from hurting someone else's feelings?

4. Am I trying to prove something to myself? Someone else?

5. Why do I want to do this? What am I hoping to gain? Is this about making me happy?

If any of my answers to these questions reveal that my desire to say yes is fueled by my perfectionism, then I lean toward saying no. You may want to do the same. The more we feed our perfectionism and validation-seeking by saying yes when we really need to say no, the more our need for external approval and validation grows. If we want to let go of our perfectionist tendencies, we have to stop feeding them.

Connect

Taking care of our emotional and mental health requires that we take a break from all the messages we're constantly bombarded with. Unless you've been living under a rock, you can't go an hour without encountering a carefully crafted magazine, television, or Internet advertisement promising you how much safer, happier, healthier, or more accepted you'll be if you purchase their product. On top of the onslaught of advertisements, we're constantly being petitioned by our family, coworkers, and peers who have their own ideas about what we "should" be doing. With all the external influence, it can be hard to distinguish our own voice from the crowd's. It can be easy to lose sight of our own beliefs and desires and just mindlessly jump through the next hoop.

This happened to me when I was in graduate school. I was in a demanding program that required lots of commitment and sacrifice. In the midst of jumping the next hurdle and checking the next requirement off my long list, I realized that I had lost myself. I became so consumed with excelling at being a graduate student that I lost touch with why I was there in the first place. I got caught up in chasing accolades and accomplishments. I bought into the goals my mentors set for me and totally abandoned my own career aspirations. I wanted the people I admired to be proud of me. Surely, following my mentors' formula for success would make me happy. If only I could just work hard and achieve their goal for me, then I'd be successful and happy. I had traded my own happiness for someone else's definition of success.

Do you ever feel like you're disconnected from who you are as a person? Have you gotten so caught up in the daily grind, searching for fulfillment and happiness in external places and people that constantly fall short? To become the highest version of yourself, you need to look inside and reconnect with who you are and what you want. To reconnect with ourselves, we need to spend time alone in silence. As spiritual teacher Ram Dass said, "The quieter you become, the more you can hear." To hear our own voice, we have to be willing to slow down, let go of all the distractions, and get quiet.

Stop Being So Critical

One of the reasons why it can be hard to stop and connect with ourselves is that we don't always have the highest opinion of ourselves, which means we may not trust our own judgment. Think back to your own experience. When you come into contact with a coworker or a neighbor you don't have the highest opinion of, how do you react? Maybe you tend to keep your distance. Or perhaps you become tense and guarded, scanning their behavior for any sign that confirms your not-so-great opinion of them. This is how we can be with ourselves when, deep down inside, we do not like ourselves.

Feeling like we don't measure up, like we're just not good enough, is so common that it might as well be woven into the fabric of the human experience. We have a tendency to set unrealistic expectations for ourselves, and when we fall short of them we beat ourselves up with verbal insults that slowly eat away at our sense of self-worth. This harsh inner voice has been labeled the inner critic. Though its intentions are to keep us safe, acceptable, and productive, just like a well-meaning doctor with a poor bedside manner, our inner critic often does a terrible job of delivering its messages. That critical voice is overly rigid and harsh, and it tries to convince us that we have to achieve certain things to be acceptable and worthy. Because an inner critic lives inside us all, when we feel like we don't measure up or we don't like ourselves it can be easy to feel, think, and act negatively toward ourselves, even to the point of emotional damage.

One way to be less critical with ourselves is to get an accurate perspective on our value as an individual. When the majority of our time is spent pointing out our shortcomings and the things we do not like about ourselves, that can become our focus. Remember, what you focus on grows. Or, as author Lysa TerKeurst says, "You steer where you stare." Let's shift our focus from our flaws to our strengths.

Instead of focusing on your failures, challenge yourself to identify your gifts and talents. Take out your notebook and make a list of your positive qualities—things you admire about yourself or attributes others have complimented you on. Read this list to yourself daily. The next time your inner critic shows up, stop it dead in its tracks. Don't allow it to take up residence in your mind. Thank your inner critic for trying to keep you safe and productive, and then steer your mind toward your gifts, talents, and positive attributes. The more often you do this, the more natural it will feel to be kind to and complimentary of yourself.

Know Your Worth

All too often we base our worth on how much money we have, what we look like, our accomplishments, and/or the type of work we do. While these may be important aspects of our identity, they do not determine our value or worth, unless we let them. You are valuable and worthy of love, respect, and a fulfilling life . . . period. You don't need to earn your worth—in fact, you can't. It came etched into the fabric of your DNA. Sometimes the traumas and hardships we experience in life can convince us that we are unworthy, that there is something irreparably wrong with us and we do not matter. These voices can be so convincing that it can be hard not to buy into them. We can even be driven to the point of hating ourselves.

When feelings of unworthiness creep in, one skill that can be essential in helping you connect to your own worth and value is to practice sending yourself well wishes. This practice is a form of meditation called Lovingkindness. You can think of Lovingkindness practice like sending a "Just Because" greeting card or text to someone you care about, expressing well wishes to them.

It can be helpful to begin this practice by closing your eyes and taking a few breaths to help yourself get in the here and now. Then, allow the breath to fade into the background of your awareness. Now bring to mind a living being who makes you feel warm and fuzzy inside. It can be a person or a pet—any living being. Now, think of some well wishes you'd like to offer them. I've suggested some phrases here, but it's really important that you choose phrases that speak to you. Say the whole phrase once and then repeat:

May you be happy.

May you be healthy.

May you be safe.

May you live with ease.

Now, release the image of the loved one you brought to mind. See if it is possible to bring an image of yourself to mind. It might be a mental image of how you look today or perhaps you can bring to mind an image of how you looked when you were younger. Now, say the same well wishes to yourself and then repeat:

May I be happy.

May I be healthy.

May I be safe.

May I live with ease.

Because of our negativity bias, it can be really hard to wish ourselves well. It can feel forced or corny at first. That's okay. Developing a kinder, more loving attitude toward yourself can take time. The key is to stick with it, no matter how you feel after practicing. Just keep going.

You'll be surprised what difference a little kindness toward yourself can make over time. Each time you practice this, jot down your thoughts and feelings in your notebook afterward. Keep track of this over time, periodically looking for slight shifts in how you think and feel about giving yourself loving-kindness. My wish for you is that, with time, you will come to believe what the Buddha said: "You yourself, as much as anybody in the entire universe, deserve your love and affection."

Accept

One of the keys to a more balanced life is accepting things as they are. Life is filled with a variety of events that we simply have no control over—including how we may feel from moment to moment. We go out to the car in the morning to drive to work, only to discover that we have a flat tire. We receive the devastating news of the loss of a loved one, or we face rejection from a job that we desperately wanted. These negative events can sometimes happen inside us, too. I'm sure many of us have had the experience of lying down after a long, tiring day only to have anxious thoughts take over our minds, ruining any hope of a restful night's sleep.

Accepting negative events, both external and internal, can save us a lot of heartache and suffering. When we resist what we are experiencing or try to make it go away, it only *intensifies* the experience. It's like trying to ignore an overly friendly pet. I am extremely allergic to cats. Anytime I visit the home of a cat owner, I avoid touching their furry friend because I know I'll pay for it later with itchy eyes and a stuffy nose. For some reason, every cat I've ever tried to avoid can sense that I'm avoiding them, and they go out of their way to get me to rub them. First, they look up at me with affectionate eyes. Then, when that doesn't work, they'll walk by me rubbing their body against my leg. If all else fails, they come sit in my lap, silently begging for my rubs and affection. I promise, this happens *all the time*. The point is, they notice that I'm trying to avoid them, but that doesn't make them go away—in fact, they come on stronger.

It's the same way with our emotions and other experiences. When we refuse to accept the reality of what's happening by fighting against it, we ultimately cause ourselves greater suffering. But please note: Acceptance is not the same thing as giving in or giving up when faced with something unpleasant. Rather, acceptance is a state of mind that says, "This is how it is. I acknowledge the reality of what's happening right now, even if I don't want or like it." Acceptance involves making a choice to not fight against what is happening. It's making a wise choice not to try to change things that are outside of our control.

Affirmations

Affirmations can help us accept the hard realities in our lives by helping us adopt an optimistic mind-set. Affirmations are statements of truth that promote inner peace, happiness, and empowerment that remind you of your full potential and give you the encouragement to live in a world that is filled with pain and uncertainty. Affirmations are *not* simply ignoring the realities of life and deluding yourself with a bunch of fake positivity. They inspire, energize, and help reconnect you with reality. Here are a few examples:

> I am enough.
>
> I have everything I need within me to achieve my goals.
>
> I choose courage.
>
> I love and approve of myself.
>
> I trust the process.

When your world feels completely unpredictable and out of control, affirmations remind you that you're capable of influencing the direction of your life—even though you can't control everything, you can control *some* things. When memories of the past start looming and try to convince you that you are damaged, affirmations can connect you with the truth: You are not defined by your past. You can control how you experience the challenges of life by speaking truth over your situation and choosing to direct your mind in a positive way.

Affirmations aren't magic. At first, they might not even be believable. Learning to be optimistic and accept things we cannot change is an inner skill that takes time to develop. To help you develop a more positive mind-set, download a free affirmation app such as ThinkUp: Positive Affirmations on your smartphone. Choose affirmations that speak to you, or create some of your own. You may want to write down the affirmations that speak to you in your notebook or use the Notes app on your smartphone. Then practice saying these truths out loud to yourself. Hint: They can be a wonderful addition to your morning routine.

Self-Compassion

When you make mistakes, what is your default response? If I were to listen in on the private conversations going on in your mind when you fall short of the expectations you have for yourself, would I hear kindness or harsh criticism? Self-compassion is another skill you can develop to help you be kind to yourself when you are experiencing emotional pain or disappointment. It involves giving yourself the same care and nurturing you would lovingly give to a toddler who has fallen down while learning to walk. To practice self-compassion, there must be a hurt or pain that needs to be soothed.

According to self-compassion researcher Kristin Neff, there are three components to self-compassion: The first component is being in the present moment—being alert and aware of what is happening in the here and now. Mindfulness helps you view the pain realistically rather than becoming consumed by it, ignoring it all together, or trying to make it "go away." The second component is recognizing that you are not alone in your pain. Emotional pain is an inevitable human experience that we all face throughout our lifetimes. Recognizing that pain is a shared human experience helps us feel less alone when we're suffering. The third component of self-compassion is self-kindness. This means being soft and gentle with yourself when you fall short of the mark, rather than being judgmental, harsh, or critical.

A simple way to begin practicing self-compassion the next time you fail or make a mistake is to talk to yourself the same way you would your best friend, child, or dear loved one when they encounter emotional pain. Use the same words, tone, and demeanor that you would use with a dear loved one toward yourself. When you struggle, meet yourself with kind understanding.

There are also many exercises online that can help you develop compassion for yourself, including writing exercises and guided imagery. A great place to start is Dr. Kristin Neff's website: www .self-compassion.org; click on Practices.

Reward Yourself

Reward yourself for prioritizing your emotional self-care by scheduling a "day date" with yourself. Fill the day with activities you enjoy. Don't worry about what others will think. Just simply schedule a day filled with things you enjoy. When the day comes, minimize distractions by letting nonessential tasks go. Fully participate in each activity you scheduled by throwing yourself 100 percent into the activity—giving it all of your energy, attention, and effort. Try your best to let go of any judgments, worries, or self-consciousness that might arise.

Grow

Taking care of ourselves emotionally can be enhanced by self-validation, gratitude, and giving ourselves permission to be flawed and imperfect. Self-validation helps us soothe and comfort ourselves when we are experiencing uncomfortable emotions. Gratitude is a practice that opens our eyes to the multitude of ways we are fortunate and blessed even though we may not be where we want to be in our lives. Gratitude promotes contentment where there is desperation and restlessness. Finally, giving yourself permission to be flawed and imperfect protects you from the heartache of consistently falling short of perfectionist standards.

Validate Yourself

We often look to others to give us the validation we can give ourselves. While support from others is incredibly important, we should be careful to not rely too heavily on others for all our emotional support. When we practice self-validation, we acknowledge our emotions and make space for them, allowing ourselves to be just as we are. We also connect our emotions to actual events, recognizing that the emotion didn't just come out of the blue, but stemmed from a real experience. We acknowledge that our emotions make sense given the circumstances from which they arose.

Validating your emotions helps you manage them effectively rather than avoiding them or trying to make them different from what they are. By acknowledging them as true and warranted given what happened, self-validation lets you off the hook for having to justify or get rid of uncomfortable emotions. Self-validation requires two steps:

1. **Identify the emotion.** For example, "I feel sad."

2. **Assert why this emotion makes sense by connecting it to an external or internal event or experience.** For example, "It makes sense that I feel sad because I just learned about the passing of a friend. Anyone would feel sad if their friend died."

These two steps may sound simple, but it may take some effort to identify how you are feeling and why you might be feeling that way. So, give yourself time to explore your answers.

Gratitude

Being thankful for what you already have helps you realize that you have more than you think. I've already talked about how relentless advertising companies can be when it comes to trying to convince us that we are not enough or don't already have enough. If we're not careful, this can lead to us spending our days and nights obsessing over how we can make more money to get more things. We can also internalize this "never enough" mentality to the point that we become perpetually unsatisfied with our lives, convinced that we need something new, better, and different in order to be happy.

Gratitude can provide peace and contentment in the midst of the daily race for different, better, and more. Not only will it help you appreciate what you have, but practicing gratitude has also been shown to improve physical and mental health, increase life satisfaction, strengthen relationships, and create a shift to a more positive perspective on negative situations. One way to build more gratitude in your life is simply to begin writing down one thing you are thankful for daily. You can dedicate a few pages in your notebook for this practice, if you'd like.

If you want to get a little creative with expressing your gratitude, consider making a "gratitude jar." Decorate a mason-style jar to your liking, cut little slips of paper, and then, each day, write one thing you are grateful for on one of the slips and place it in the jar. Make a habit of this activity by adding at least one item to the jar at the same time each day.

Committed Action: Take Responsibility for Your Emotions

You've learned that we can't necessarily control our emotions; we cannot simply will ourselves to feel a different way. However, we can take intentional, committed actions that move us closer to our goals. Instead of sitting on the sidelines of our life hoping that we'll feel better "one day," we can take intentional action to help boost our mood. For example, if you're feeling sad, you can listen to music that uplifts your spirits, or read books that help you feel hopeful.

There are other, bigger actions we can take toward our goals. If we recognize that we need better coping strategies, we can seek out therapy. When we're feeling lonely, we can reach out to supportive friends. When I am in the midst of a disagreement with a loved one, rather than lashing out in hurt and anger I can choose to express my emotions calmly. When I am feeling frustrated or disappointed, rather than bottling up my feelings I can express them through journaling.

No matter what emotions come your way, you always have the choice of how you will respond. When challenging emotions arise, let your response be guided by the responses you listed in the "What

Relationship Do You Want to Have with Your Feelings?" exercise (see page 111). Look over your responses. It is likely that developing this relationship with your emotions will require you to be willing to experience uncomfortable thoughts, feelings, sensations, and urges.

In your notebook, write down the thoughts, feelings, sensations, and urges you are willing to have in order to develop a healthier relationship with your emotions. What small step can you take to begin cultivating this relationship?

Chapter Highlights

- Emotional self-care involves acknowledging and embracing all your emotions—the pleasant feelings and the unpleasant feelings—and giving yourself what you need.
- When you have an assertive relationship with your emotions, although you cannot control them, you recognize that you have the power to influence your feelings. You know, ultimately, that you control how you respond when feeling emotional, and you take the initiative to set your environment up in a way that helps you cope effectively.
- Learning how to say no is not only a good time-management strategy, but it also nurtures your emotional health by ensuring that you are spending your precious time engaged in the activities that are most important and valuable to you.
- When you resist what you are experiencing or try to make it go away, it only intensifies the experience.
- Taking care of yourself emotionally can be enhanced by self-validation, gratitude, and giving yourself permission to be flawed and imperfect.

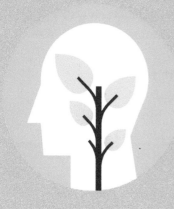

CHAPTER 8

Self-Care
A Prescription for Living

Building the Self-Care Habit

Congratulations! You've done a lot of work on your journey through this book, and hopefully you're already seeing some of the many benefits that come with taking better care of *you*. Thank you for allowing me to be a part of your self-care journey. Most important, you deserve a huge round of applause for taking this step. Just the fact that you read this book is evidence that you not only care about yourself, but you are also actively taking steps to become an all-around healthier and happier person. Seriously, THIS IS A BIG DEAL. So many people spend the majority of their lives on autopilot—just existing but not truly living a life they enjoy.

Now's the time to start thinking about what you will take away from this experience to help you sustain the gains you made on your self-care journey. As you know, this book covered a lot of material. You shouldn't expect—or even try—to remember every exercise, tip, and strategy. I encourage you to thumb through the pages of this book and your notebook and review the new skills, insights, and ideas you gained while making your way through the book.

What resonated most with you? What were your favorite takeaways? What didn't seem to fit for you? Because we are more likely to retain information when we break it down into manageable slices, I'm going to suggest that you flip to the next page in your notebook and generate a list of your two favorite takeaways from each chapter. Be sure to write down things you can imagine integrating into your routine.

Building habits takes time. Wouldn't it be nice if we could just program ourselves like robots to automatically take up new habits without the burden of self-discipline, consistency, or practice? Unfortunately, our human minds can't be programmed the way we program our computers. We need to practice new habits to make them stick. To make your new self-care routines second nature, you will need self-discipline, consistency, and practice.

When we get excited about building new healthy habits, it can be tempting to try to change everything all at once. It is easy to get super motivated and unknowingly set yourself up for failure by trying to implement too much change too soon. I invite you to start simple. Of the five domains of self-care, choose one domain to focus on initially and then build up from that. For instance, if you want to start with physical self-care, focus only on implementing one new physical self-care activity for a solid month. At the end of the month, consider adding one self-care activity from that same domain or another. Continuing to gradually build in this way will give you the best chance of creating strong self-care habits.

Personalizing Your Routine

The ancient Greek philosopher Heraclitus once said "Change is the only constant in life." This quote reminds us that change is inevitable. Just as the weather changes from day to day and each year we progress through four seasons, our bodies, perspectives, and needs regularly change—sometimes day to day. It follows that our self-care needs will change, too. Knowing this, we need to be ready to embrace that change.

One thing you can do to stay on track with your changing needs is check in with yourself regularly. Stop, if only for a moment, get quiet, and tune in to your body. Connect with your breath. Feel the rise and fall of your belly as you breathe in and out. Simply notice what thoughts are running through your head without trying to change them or make them go away. Put your hand on your chest. Feel the strong and steady thump of your heart beating against your chest. Sense the temperature on your skin. Just like you are intentional about staying in contact with close friends or relatives, stay in touch with yourself.

Make a commitment to spend a little time in silence with yourself at least once a week, even if it's only five minutes. It may even be helpful to make this a morning routine. During this time, take out your notebook. Start by asking yourself three questions:

1. How am I feeling right now?

2. What do I need in this moment?

3. What small action can I take to feed my soul today?

Pause. Listen for the answer. Then let the pen effortlessly release your thoughts onto the page. This is a no-judgment zone: there's no second-guessing or guilt allowed. Simply let the pen become an instrument of your heart, gently releasing the wisdom and guidance that lies within you.

Make an honest assessment of how much time you are spending doing things that nurture you. When you notice that you're out of balance, don't beat yourself up; just make adjustments as necessary. Keep using the skills you've learned while reading this book. If one skill stops working for you, try another. Keep adjusting your self-care routine in this way to suit your evolving needs. Choosing self-care is not always easy, but I believe you can do hard things. You have the power within you to choose and create your reality.

Walking the Path to Wellness

This is where the first part of our journey together ends, my friend—though I hope that you will return to this book many times in the future for support. I'm so grateful you took this ride with me. Remember, keeping your life in balance is an ongoing journey. By making time for yourself, getting in touch with what matters most to you, setting priorities, and showing up for your life in new ways, you have the resources you need to make self-care a habit for a lifetime. It's not a sprint. Just keep jogging. You may need to stop a time or two to catch your breath and modify your strategy. That's okay. When you're ready, get back in the race. As author and thought leader Tony Robbins says, "Stay committed to your decisions, but stay flexible in your approach." Stay committed to this lifelong journey of self-care. I'm right alongside you, jogging in my own self-care lane, cheering for you. You've got this!

More Resources

If you want more support to help keep you going along your self-care journey, check out these resources.

Books

I seriously cannot say enough about how much treasure can be found in books! Not only is reading essential for intellectual self-care, it is an excellent way to get inspiration and encouragement for all the domains of self-care as well. Here are some of my favorite self-care books:

- *Daring Greatly: How the Courage to Be Vulnerable Transforms the Way We Live, Love, Parent, and Lead* by Brené Brown
- *The Gifts of Imperfection: Let Go of Who You Think You're Supposed to Be and Embrace Who You Are* by Brené Brown
- *I Thought It Was Just Me (but it isn't): Making the Journey from "What Will People Think?" to "I Am Enough"* by Brené Brown
- *On Fire: The 7 Choices to Ignite a Radically Inspired Life* by John O' Leary
- *You Are a Badass: How to Stop Doubting Your Greatness and Start Living an Awesome Life* by Jen Sincero

I also love to read memoirs and spiritual texts for inspiration, spiritual fulfillment, and a fresh perspective on life. Some of my favorites are:

- *Becoming* by Michelle Obama
- *Breathe: Making Room for Sabbath* by Priscilla Shirer
- *Don't Settle for Safe: Embracing the Uncomfortable to Become Unstoppable* by Sarah Jakes Roberts
- *5 Habits of a Woman Who Doesn't Quit* by Nicki Koziarz
- *Why Her?: 6 Truths We Need to Hear When Measuring Up Leaves Us Falling Behind* by Nicki Koziarz
- *It's Not Supposed to Be This Way: Finding Unexpected Strength When Disappointments Leave You Shattered* by Lysa TerKeurst
- *Make Your Move: Finding Unshakable Confidence Despite Your Fears and Failures* by Lynn Cowell
- *The Book of Awakening: Having the Life You Want by Being Present to the Life You Have* by Mark Nepo

Apps

I have found apps to be a useful and convenient way to help keep me accountable and provide new ways of practicing physical, intellectual, spiritual, and emotional self-care. Here are just a few of my favorites: Insight Timer, Calm, ThinkUp, Bible, First 5 by Proverbs 31 Ministry, Five Minute Journal, MyFitnessPal, and C25K.

Websites

The Internet is full of free resources that can give you ideas about self-care and ways to engage in self-care. If you are interested in practicing mindfulness, one rich resource is the University of California Center for Mindfulness: https://health.ucsd.edu /specialties/mindfulness/

Another website I mentioned earlier as a good resource for a progressive muscle relaxation exercise is Dartmouth Student Wellness Center. You can access it free of charge here: https://students .dartmouth.edu/wellness-center/wellness-mindfulness/relaxation -downloads/progressive-muscle-relaxation

These are just two examples of the material you can find on the Internet. Do your research to find resources that can support you in the various domains of self-care you would like to improve.

Online Communities

One of the positive aspects of social media is that you can connect with people from across the world who share your values. Facebook groups can be a fantastic way to build connections and support your self-care in a variety of domains. Whether you are looking for accountability, advice, or new ways to spice up your exercise routine, you can find a Facebook group for it. Aside from social media, many of today's thought leaders, such as Brené Brown, have e-mail lists you can join if you'd like to receive weekly encouragement and inspiration. The next time you're online, keep an eye out for communities you can join to support you along your self-care journey.

Therapy

Sometimes you just need an outsider's perspective, someone who is unbiased and trained to help you manage the challenges you're facing. Therapy is one of the best gifts you can give yourself. It is often covered by insurance, so you can take care of *you* without fears of breaking the bank! If therapy is not covered in your current policy, talk to your doctor about community mental health options that might be available. I cannot stress enough how important it is to do your research and find a therapist who is a good fit for you. You could potentially be delving into really personal and private topics. You want to do that with someone you feel comfortable with.

To ensure that they have the training, experience, and knowledge to help you navigate your unique challenges, it is important to check out the expertise of a particular therapist you are interested in. For instance, if you are struggling to manage anxiety, you want to select a therapist who has a proven track record of helping their clients better manage anxiety. You are entrusting this person with your mental health, so you want to make sure they provide high-quality and culturally competent services.

Your therapist should be someone who fits your personality and preferences. Because fit with a therapist is so important, you should know that it may take you a few tries to find the right therapist for you. Don't get discouraged if you don't connect with the first person you see. Some good websites that can assist you in choosing the right therapist for you are:

- American Association of Christian Counselors: www.aacc.net
- American Psychological Association Psychologist Locator: locator.apa.org
- Find a Psychologist: www.findapsychologist.org
- Psychology Today: www.psychologytoday.com
- Therapy for Black Girls Therapist Directory: www.therapyforblackgirls .com/therapist-directory

References

Adkins, Amy. "Employee Engagement in U.S. Stagnant in 2015." *Gallup.* January 13, 2016. news.gallup.com/poll/188144/employee-engagement-stagnant-2015.aspx.

Ajiboye, Tolu. "Adults Need Recess Too. Here's Why You Should Make Time to Play." *NBC News.* July 7, 2018. www.nbcnews.com/better/health/adults-need-recess-too-here-s-why-you-should-make-ncna887396.

Bateson, Patrick, and Paul Martin. *Play, Playfulness, Creativity and Innovation.* Cambridge: Cambridge University Press, 2013.

Baumeister, Roy F., and Mark R. Leary. "The Need to Belong: Desire for Interpersonal Attachments as a Fundamental Human Motivation." *Psychological Bulletin* 117, no. 3 (May 1995): 497–529. https://doi.org/10.1037/0033-2909.117.3.497.

Cohen, Sheldon. "Social Relationships and Health." *American Psychologist* 59, no. 8 (November 2004): 676–84. https://dx.doi.org/10.1037/0003-066X.59.8.676.

Costello, Peter C. *Attachment-Based Psychotherapy: Helping Patients Develop Adaptive Capacities.* Washington, DC: American Psychological Association, 2013.

Fredrickson, Barbara L., Michael A. Cohn, Kimberly A. Coffey, Jolynn Pek, and Sandra M. Finkel. "Open Hearts Build Lives: Positive Emotions, Induced Through Loving-Kindness Meditation, Build Consequential Personal Resources." *Journal of Personality and Social Psychology* 95, no. 5 (November 2008): 1045–62. https://doi.org/10.1037/a0013262.

Galloway, Ann P., and Melissa Henry. "Relationships Between Social Connectedness and Spirituality and Depression and Perceived Health Status of Rural Residents." *Online Journal of Rural Nursing & Health Care* 14, no. 2 (October 2014): 43–79. https://doi.org/10.14574/ojrnhc.v14i2.325.

Gottman, John Mordechai, and Nan Silver. *The Seven Principles for Making Marriage Work: A Practical Guide from the Country's Foremost Relationship Expert.* rev. ed. New York: Harmony, 2015.

Harvard Men's Health Watch. "Exercising to Relax." Updated July 13, 2018. www.health.harvard.edu/staying-healthy/exercising-to-relax.

Hirshkowitz, Max, Kaitlyn Whiton, Steven M. Albert, Cathy Alessi, Oliviero Bruni, Lydia DonCarlos, Nancy Hazen, et al. "National Sleep Foundation's Sleep Time Duration Recommendations: Methodology and Results Summary." *Sleep Health Journal* 1, no. 1 (March 2015): 40–43. https://doi.org/10.1016/j.sleh.2014.12.010.

Jiang, Da, Diane Hosking, Richard Burns, and Kaarin J. Anstey. "Volunteering Benefits Life Satisfaction Over 4 Years: The Moderating Role of Social Network Size." *Australian Journal of Psychology* 70, no. 3 (August 2018). https://doi.org/10.1111/ajpy.12217.

Kabat-Zinn, Jon. "An Outpatient Program in Behavioral Medicine for Chronic Pain Patients Based on the Practice of Mindfulness Meditation: Theoretical Considerations and Preliminary Results." *General Hospital Psychiatry* 4, no. 1 (April 1982): 33–42. https://doi.org/10.1016/0163-8343(82)90026-3.

Kabat–Zinn, Jon. "Mindfulness–Based Interventions in Context: Past, Present, and Future." *Clinical Psychology: Science and Practice* 10, no. 2 (May 2006): 144–56. https://doi.org/10.1093/clipsy.bpg016.

Lee, Richard M., Matthew Draper, and Sujin Lee. "Social Connectedness, Dysfunctional Interpersonal Behaviors, and Psychological Distress: Testing a Mediator Model." *Journal of Counseling Psychology* 48, no. 3 (July 2001): 310–18. http://dx.doi.org/10.1037/0022-0167.48.3.310.

Maslow, A. H. "A Theory of Human Motivation." *Psychological Review* 50, no. 4 (1943): 370-96. psychclassics.yorku.ca/Maslow/motivation.htm.

National Eating Disorders Alliance. "Body Image and Eating Disorders." Accessed March 15, 2019. www.nationaleatingdisorders.org/body-image-eating-disorders.

National Heart, Lung, and Blood Institute. "Physical Activity and Your Heart." Accessed March 15, 2019. www.nhlbi.nih.gov/health-topics/physical-activity-and-your-heart.

National Institute on Aging. "Participating in Activities You Enjoy." Reviewed October 23, 2017. Accessed March 15, 2019. www.nia.nih.gov/health/participating-activities-you-enjoy.

National Wellness Institute. "The Six Dimensions of Wellness." Accessed May 2, 2019. https://www.nationalwellness.org/page/Six_Dimensions.

Neff, Kristin. "Definition of Self-Compassion." Accessed May 2, 2019. https://self-compassion.org/the-three-elements-of-self-compassion-2/.

Piliavin, Jane Allyn, and Erica Siegl. "Health Benefits of Volunteering in the Wisconsin Longitudinal Study." *Journal of Health and Social Behavior* 48, no. 4 (December 2007): 450–64. https://doi.org/10.1177/002214650704800408.

Ratcliff, Roger, and Hans P.A. Van Dongen. "The Effects of Sleep Deprivation on Item and Associative Recognition Memory." *Journal of Experimental Psychology: Learning, Memory, and Cognition* 44, no. 2 (February 2018): 193–208. https://doi.org/10.1037/xlm0000452.

Rubinstein, Joshua S., David E. Meyer, and Jeffrey E. Evans. "Executive Control of Cognitive Processes in Task Switching." *Journal of Experimental Psychology: Human Perception and Performance* 27, no. 4 (August 2001): 763–97. http://dx.doi.org/10.1037/0096-1523.27.4.763.

Salzberg, Sharon. *Lovingkindness: The Revolutionary Art of Happiness.* Boulder, CO: Shambhala, 1995.

Segal, Zindel V., J. Mark G. Williams, and John D. Teasdale. *Mindfulness-Based Cognitive Therapy for Depression: A New Approach to Preventing Relapse.* New York: Guilford Press, 2001.

Sidani, Jaime E., Ariel Shensa, Beth Hoffman, Janel Hanmer, and Brian A. Primack. "The Association Between Social Media Use and Eating Concerns Among US Young Adults." *Journal of the Academy of Nutrition and Dietetics* 116, no. 9 (September 2016): 1465–72. https://doi.org/10.1016/j.jand.2016.03.021.

Spangler, Todd. "Are Americans Addicted to Smartphones? U.S. Consumers Check Their Phones 52 Times Daily, Study Finds." *Variety.* November 14, 2018. variety.com/2018/digital/news/smartphone-addiction-study-check-phones-52-times-daily1203028454/.

Steiner, Susie. "Top Five Regrets of the Dying." *The Guardian.* February 1, 2012. www.theguardian.com/lifeandstyle/2012/feb/01/top-five-regrets-of-the-dying.

Teasdale, John, Mark Williams, and Zindel V. Segal. *The Mindful Way Workbook: An 8-Week Program to Free Yourself from Depression and Emotional Distress.* New York: Guilford Press, 2014.

TerKeurst, Lysa. *It's Not Supposed to Be This Way: Finding Unexpected Strength When Disappointments Leave You Shattered.* Nashville, TN: Thomas Nelson, 2018.

US Department of Agriculture. "MyPlate Plan." January 2016. https://choosemyplate-prod.azureedge.net/sites/default/files/myplate/checklists/MyPlatePlan_2000cals_Age14plus.pdf.

US Department of Health and Human Services. "Executive Summary: Physical Activity Guidelines for Americans, 2nd edition." Accessed March 15, 2019. health.gov/paguidelines/second-edition/pdf/PAG_ExecutiveSummary.pdf.

Voelker, Dana K., Justine J. Reel, and Christy Greenleaf. "Weight Status and Body Image Perceptions in Adolescents: Current Perspectives." *Adolescent Health, Medicine and Therapeutics* 6 (August 2015): 149–58. https://doi.org/10.2147/AHMT.S68344.

Willcox, Gloria. "The Feeling Wheel: A Tool for Expanding Awareness of Emotions and Increasing Spontaneity and Intimacy." *Transactional Analysis Journal* 12, no. 4 (1982): 274–76. http://dx.doi.org/10.1177/036215378201200411.

Index

About the Author

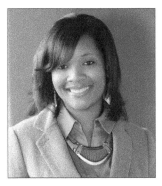

Robyn L. Gobin, PhD, is a licensed clinical psychologist, mindfulness instructor, speaker, researcher, and university professor. Propelled by her values of faith and making a difference, Robyn has an unrelenting focus on helping others improve their lives by taking charge of their thoughts and embracing their worth. Witnessing the shame, silence, and lack of mental health knowledge in the Black church during her childhood sparked Robyn's desire to improve well-being in the larger Black community. To positively impact her community, Robyn earned her master's and PhD in clinical psychology from the University of Oregon.

A trauma psychologist specializing in women's mental health and ethnically diverse populations, Robyn enjoys helping survivors of sexual violence reclaim their lives. Her research aims to alleviate pain and suffering among diverse trauma survivors, including U.S. military veterans. She has served on numerous boards and committees for mental health and nonprofit organizations, and actively presents and publishes her work.

In addition to her professional interests, Robyn is committed to reducing stigma and shame surrounding mental health issues in the Black community. Robyn enjoys speaking at women's conferences and facilitating retreats and workshops where she explores how mental and spiritual principles can be combined to manage life's challenges. Robyn was recently awarded a Citizen Psychologist Citation from the President of the American Psychological Association for her leadership in reducing barriers to mental health treatment for ethnic minority populations and creating an educational pipeline for the next generation of culturally diverse leaders in the field of psychology. Robyn is the proud wife of Korey and adoring mother to Justice, her four-legged son. In her free time, Robyn enjoys snuggling on the couch with her family for movie night, reading for spiritual nourishment, and trying new recipes.

CPSIA information can be obtained
at www.ICGtesting.com
Printed in the USA
JSHW021912240220
4423JS00004B/4